A Year of Days

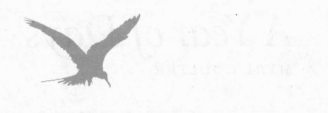

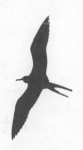

A Year of Days

MYRL COULTER

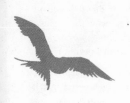

 The University of Alberta Press

Published by

The University of Alberta Press
Ring House 2
Edmonton, Alberta, Canada T6G 2E1
www.uap.ualberta.ca

Copyright © 2015 Myrl Coulter

Library and Archives Canada Cataloguing in Publication

Coulter, Myrl, author
    A year of days / Myrl Coulter.

(Robert Kroetsch series)
Issued in print and electronic formats.
ISBN 978-1-77212-045-5 (pbk.).—ISBN 978-1-77212-078-3 (epub).—
ISBN 978-1-77212-079-0 (kindle).—ISBN 978-1-77212-080-6 (pdf)

    I. Title. II. Series: Robert Kroetsch series

PS8605.O8935Y43 2015   C814'.6   C2014-908311-4   C2014-908312-2

First edition, first printing, 2015.
Printed and bound in Canada by Houghton Boston Printers, Saskatoon,
Saskatchewan.
Copyediting and proofreading by Helen Moffett.

A volume in the Robert Kroetsch Series.

The University of Alberta Press gratefully acknowledges the support
received for its publishing program from The Canada Council for the Arts.
The University of Alberta Press also gratefully acknowledges the financial
support of the Government of Canada through the Canada Book Fund (CBF)
and the Government of Alberta through the Alberta Media Fund (AMF) for
its publishing activities.

Canada   Canada Council   Conseil des Arts   Alberta
            for the Arts   du Canada   Government

For Mom

into the cirrus-drift of age—
those faint streaks that trail after grief,
remembering its passage.

– Alice Major, *Memory's Daughter*

Contents

Gut Feelings

When I was a child, I sometimes felt an uncontrollable urge to laugh at the worst possible moment, perhaps during a sermon in church, or when my parents were giving me a stern talking-to. The feeling would start in my belly and silently bubble its way up to my mouth. The more I tried to hold it in, the more it refused to co-operate, the more it demanded a vocal exit. It would come out as a laugh—a weak tentative one, but a laugh nonetheless. I'd hear those dreaded words from the authority figures around me: "You think this is funny?" I'd struggle to regain my solemn face and shake my lowering head. The rising anxiety in my gut prevented me from finding the words to say that no, I didn't think it was funny, and yes, I knew the situation was serious. Later, I would mull over my irrepressible, ill-advised laughter. What the heck was wrong with me?

Laughing is a form of stress release, no matter what the source is. Nervous or tentative laughter is often a response to tension and anxiety. For the younger me, my awkward events occurred in moments of conflict, when my body's emotional state revolved around what would happen next. My inappropriate laughter usually came when I wanted to run, maybe during an intense family discussion, or in an attempt to shield myself in a situation of my own making—an instinctive, fruitless effort to escape the consequences of skipping school or sassing my mother. The much older me knows now that this kind of laughter is an involuntary reaction, one that comes from discomfort or confusion or fear, almost any negative emotion— anything but humour. I wish I'd known that when I was ten.

Much of my emotional life has reflected those involuntary outbursts of laughter, those escaped responses born of my viscerality. Viscerality is not an official word. It's not listed in any dictionary that I've seen. But whether it officially exists or not doesn't matter to me. I like the way its five syllables run together, the way my mouth has to shape and reshape itself to say it. I like it, so I use it. Viscerality comes from words that do exist in official dictionaries, root cousins such as the adjective "visceral" and the noun "viscera." It is a re-nouned noun. Adding the suffix "ity" onto the root noun's adjective changes "visceral" from a descriptive back into a defined condition. Viscerality is a condition I know well.

The *Oxford English Dictionary* defines "viscera" as referring to the bowels. This venerable tome also notes that the bowels are "the seat of emotion." The gut. Our guts are viscera, visceral, the viscerality of our very existence, where we feel what we eat and eat what we feel. These days I feel the condition of my viscerality more than I used to, and it makes me anxious, almost to the point of inappropriate laughter.

Anxiety also makes me nauseous. "In through the nose, out through the mouth" is a mantra I've used for years, ever since a now-nameless doctor advised me that this technique would help me manage my frequent bouts of nausea, or at least delay vomiting until I got myself to a proper upchucking place, like a bathroom or a garage. Nausea is something I've become very familiar with over the years. It's the go-to symptom for my body. If some disturbance looms, whether from an incoming bout of flu or a looming oral dissertation exam, the first symptom I'm likely to feel is nausea.

Nausea is the reason I gave up on carnival rides early in my life. Back in my hometown of Winnipeg, I went to the Red River Exhibition every June. As a teenager on a date with a boy I wanted to impress, I feigned a happy anticipation for all the exciting rides ahead of us that evening. "Yes, of course I love rides," I said. "Can't get enough of them." I made it through three. The last one was something called the "Wild Mouse," where we sat huddled in a mouse-shaped car that hurtled around far too many hairpin turns. When the ride finally ended, I got out on very wobbly legs, staggered down the ramp, and threw up behind the ticket booth. I still don't know whether I was puking from fear or candy floss.

Like nausea, embarrassment is visceral. This I know for certain. What I don't know is why people turn red when they're embarrassed. I'm aware of the anatomical reasons; I know that the flush is caused by an adrenalin rush released by our instinct to flee, that a rise in blood pressure results from that rush. It puzzles me nonetheless. I don't doubt the science, but I think there has to be more to it than that. Years ago, my teenaged face turned red if I burped out loud while answering a question during English class or farted while doing calisthenics in Phys Ed. I'd look around to see if anyone noticed. Then I'd cover my face until the redness faded. Now much older, less inclined to be embarrassed about gas escaping from my body, and more prone to moments when my inside voice refuses to be contained, I am ever more curious about the physical symptoms of emotion, whether they're rendered as stoic silence or impulsive reflex.

We often think of our emotional signals as coming from the heart, but we know they don't. Our hearts are muscles.

They are fluid pumps, not management centres for laughing or crying. When I laugh out loud at my toddler grandson's antics, or gasp when I see a cyclist almost get hit by a car, or sob in my bathroom because this freaking world can sometimes be a lonely place, my brain is busy working. In the moment's heat, I don't care that my physical emotional response began in my brain stem, in the limbic area, in my hypothalamus region, which I can't see, located as it is in the middle of my head, at a level somewhere below my eyebrows and above my ears.

When I watch a violent scene in a movie, I feel it in my gut—although less so if the movie is mediocre and I don't care about the characters. In that case, I eat my trans fat infused popcorn and evaluate the choreographed action. But if I'm invested in the story, and a character I've grown to care about is threatened, I feel physical symptoms. They manifest themselves as shortness of breath or a broad ache that spreads through my abdomen. If the scene is prolonged, both my arms start to tingle right down to my hands. I begin to sweat. If the situation intensifies, my legs get restless. Then my throat squinches, making me feel like I want to swallow, but can't, because my shortness of breath has turned into hyperventilation. By this point, my viscerality has completely taken me over.

I like New Year's Day. The idea of starting again every fifty-two weeks, of setting the calendar back to the beginning, has great appeal for me. I've come to relish the calm quiet of the year's first day. The lazy couch time is as enjoyable for me as the celebration the night before. In my life, I've had my share of New Year's Eve hoopla, of parties and hats and noisemakers and champagne—well, maybe I haven't quite had my full share of champagne yet. I've spent New Year's Eve at fancy dress balls, sit-down dinners, Chinese restaurants, outdoor concerts, and even one moonlit skating party where we sailed down a frozen creek fortified by hot chocolate laced with Bailey's Irish Cream. I've also had very quiet New Years' Eves, nights when I was unable to keep my eyes open long enough to celebrate the old man turning into a diapered baby.

And despite its weather, I have some affection for the month of January. I like its relative calm. It's a month for thinking rather than feeling, for thinking about feeling. Thinking about feelings is hard work. January work. Most readily accomplished in a muffled environment. When I wake up on the first day of the first month of the fresh year, I don't make any resolutions. I gave up on that self-imposed pressure years ago. Why spend time making impossible promises to myself? What I do instead is think. Long slow thoughts. I've learned that I need to take the first few weeks of the year to think about what comes next. I've also learned not to be hard on myself if this thinking takes more than a few weeks, or takes more than a month, or even takes a whole year of days.

In our crowded contemporary calendar, holidays are multi-tasking events. They are official or unofficial. They serve religious or secular, national or international, individual or communal purposes. They are specifically cultural or expansively inclusive. What they mean to most people is a day off work.

I grew curious about what else our major holidays mean, what their roots are, and why they appear on our calendars year after year. I began a casual investigation, during which I stumbled across a few special occasions I'd like to add to my year. In September, there's International Talk-Like-a-Pirate Day. And there's something called Mole Day on October twenty-third. I was intrigued until I realized that Mole Day does not celebrate the animal or the Mexican sauce, but a unit of chemical measure. It's a day for chemists, which I am definitely not. My preferred periodic table is a punctuation chart. But I like the sounds of the very rare Square Root Day, which happens only nine times a century. And then there's Belly Laugh Day, which happens on the twenty-fourth of January. I think I'll start celebrating Belly Laugh Day. Just saying it out loud makes me want to chuckle.

But those days are unique in their obscure eccentricity, lost in the loudness of the more popular annual markers. Every year, restaurants and flower shops promote love on Valentine's Day by raising their prices. Every year, single people around the world sit apart from the hat-wearing, Chinese-food-eating, champagne-popping parties of New Year's Eve, the loneliest night of the year for the person sitting in front of a television set with an empty bowl of popcorn and a beer. Many times each year, cheery greetings tell us what we're supposed to feel: Happy Birthday, Happy Easter, Happy Halloween, Happy Canada Day, Happy Mother's/Father's/St. Patrick's Day. Happy, happy, happy. It's a constant command. For many, that mandated happiness is a heavy façade, a shroud to hide anxiety, loneliness, sadness, despair, anger.

The days of each year, special and otherwise, speed by and I wonder why we are so eager to get to the next one. Why do we rush to anticipate the highlights of each month, season, year? "I can't wait until..." is a common way to begin a sentence or a conversation. We wish our ordinary days away, throw ourselves into tomorrow, leap from one highlight day to another.

In recent years, I noticed that I'd lost that positive visceral sense of anticipation ascending from my abdomen as celebrated occasions approached. In fact, nowadays special occasions often leave me without any emotion at all. Many times, I'd prefer to ignore them, render them ordinary. Approaching biggies—Christmas, Thanksgiving, Easter—make my anxiety levels soar. Multiple questions nag at me: Why do I feel this way? What is the difference between an ordinary day and a special day? As we get older, do they switch? Do the ordinary days take on special status? Does the lustre of those special days dim? What types of conversations do our older selves have with our younger selves?

My younger self revered life and feared death. My older self still reveres life and still fears death, but not as much as it fears my life will end before I'm finished living it. And when that day does come, how do I know that I've made enough of me available to my children that they don't have to go looking for me after I'm gone?

All my life, despite those childhood outbursts of inappropriate laughter, I've thought of myself as a person who controlled her emotions very well. I didn't worry too much about what others thought. That was my version of me. But in the last few years, I noticed that I felt more emotion and was less capable of managing that emotion. Small incidents I used to shed with relative ease took a deeper hold on me. I'd find myself shaking with anger when someone cut me off on the road. Or my eyes would fill with tears at the sight of an elderly couple walking down the street holding hands. I began to think about what emotion was, where it came from, and how my feelings were subject to change as the same days rolled by again and again.

Initially associated with public upheavals such as civic uprisings, the noun "emotion" came to the English language from French. It's an umbrella noun, a fluid three-syllable collective word, abstract in the sense that what it signifies cannot be touched. Unlike trees or rocks, emotions are generally intangible. We cannot reach out and feel them with our fingertips, such as when we shop for tomatoes or weed a garden. For the most part, emotions are abstract entities. Yet, if we remember the last sobbing child we held in our arms, we realize that there are times when physical contact with someone else's feelings is possible.

In general, I am a happy person. Lucky and grateful for the privileges the accident of my birth bestowed on me. Indebted to the people who came into my life, saw my flaws, and stayed anyway. Emotion comes quickly to my surface these days, often invoked by odd sources that used to leave my younger self unaffected. In theatres or sports events or concert halls, the playing of Canada's national anthem—or almost any national anthem—brings a familiar rise of feeling from somewhere deep in my body, down near where my appendix used to be. I remain dry-eyed at the weepiest movie, but a few bars of "O Canada" has me welling up like a child denied a puppy.

In safe environments, I express my emotions. In unsafe environments, I tend to hide, suppress, deny, or ignore them. Predictably, this effort is often unsuccessful. Although emotions are largely invisible on the skin, they do show on the skin of the face and certainly on the skin of my face. I've found it quite discomfiting to discover that my emotions can move my facial muscles without my permission. Some movement is essential to emotion. Movement is contained in emotion's ether, its very structure. Movement is present in emotion's etymology, along with motivation. Emotion, movement, and motivation live inside each other.

I am not an expert in emotion. I have no neurological or psychological training in how our bodies and our brains and our emotions are connected. Facing an avalanche of wide-ranging feelings after my mother's death a few years ago, I decided to put their chaotic presence in a manageable order. I wanted to organize them, find a place to store each one.

One of my favourite rooms in my house is what I call our dressing room, an elegant moniker for a less-than-elegant space. It's a converted small bedroom, its walls tricked out with contemporary white closet organizers. My husband's clothes are on one side, mine on the other. In the middle is the ironing board, where our fancy European-style iron sits ready for use. My husband bought it. It's all steam and no heat. I don't use it. I don't know how, and I refuse to read the instructions. I don't need to because I no longer buy clothes that require ironing. But I do like watching my husband iron his shirt for the day each morning while I'm lying in bed, staying out of his way until he leaves for the office. That iron makes me smile whenever I look at it.

One day, not long after my mother died, I stood re-organizing my side of the dressing room. Looking at the clean white rails and basket drawers, I realized that this was what I wanted for my unmanageable throng of emotions. In the long section, I could hang the biggies, the ones that needed the most space: sadness, grief, rage. Contained there, they wouldn't reach out and contaminate the others. I'd also have a short section, a snappy little area where I could hang contentment and joy alongside satisfaction and happiness, an initially compact section with much room for growth. Nearby, I'd fill some of the sleek sliding wire baskets with those pesky cluttering accessories—envy, pride, and worry.

Later that morning, I went into another favourite room, again a small bedroom we converted into my office. The walls are deep sky blue. I sat down in front of my computer and searched for information on how to classify emotions. Wrapped in the burgundy writing shawl I keep on the back of my chair, I discovered that any attempt to organize human feelings into a taxonomic hierarchy is an exercise in confusion. Several websites provided charts that plotted out human emotions. Some featured smiley faces and colourful pies divided into six slices: red for anger, blue for sadness, yellow for fear, green for joy, gold for excitement, purple for passion. Some included happiness, surprise, and disgust in their emotional categories. Others had fear and remorse taking up pieces of their pies. Still others ranked feelings such as apathy, contempt, and wonder as sub-emotions. It was list chaos.

I printed many pages and spread them out around me, ready to put them into neat piles. I wanted order. Hours later, the piles were a mess, with no order in sight. So I threw all the piles into one big heap, went to my kitchen, and started a new list on a fresh sheet of paper. I wrote out the alphabet and tried to find at least one emotion for each letter. Was quizzical an emotion? What about zeal? Then I made two columns, with the headings "major" and "minor." As I listed items first in one column and then the other, I heard lyrics in my head from an old Cole Porter song: "how strange the change from major to minor." Under the major column, I had anger, fear, joy, and sadness. What about love, said a voice in my head. You have to include love on the major side. It's right there, I said to the air. It's contained in joy. No way, the air argued back. Joy isn't the same as love. Is it?

As I looked at my lists, I thought about how my body experiences each word. The majors are hard-felt and quick to strike, a collision, perhaps a hit-and-run. The minors move in with subtlety, wear disguises, and stay longer. Some of the minors are more like moods. Moods, I decided, have more artifice. They slide in as sleights, last longer than major emotional hits, but leave fewer psychic scars.

What about loneliness, asked the voice that wouldn't leave me be. I scoffed at it. Loneliness doesn't make any list. It's not an emotion or a mood, I reasoned with myself as I sat by myself. Like viscerality, loneliness is a condition, correctable with effort, perhaps correctable with love. Isn't it? It should be.

In recent years, scholastic thinkers and curious writers have delved into the links between our brains and our emotions.

Their readers are now familiar with the concept of "Emotional Intelligence," an awareness of the delicate balance between our actions and our feelings. They also know that we have "Emotional Lives" and our personalities have "Emotional Styles." These books allow us to spend time testing ourselves, administering self-quizzes, adding up our points, and applying emotional labels to our psyches.

I'm not a regular reader of self-help books, so going through these was a new experience. The child in me always feels good when I do well on tests, so I got out my pencil and fresh sheets of paper. Afterwards, I studied the results. My scores put me narrowly into the top fifty percentile when it came to resilience. I scored much higher in the areas of social intuition and self-awareness. My results revealed that I needed to work towards balancing my slightly depleted emotional stamina with my somewhat suspicious, albeit still positive, outlook.

This information in hand, I set out to use it. Perhaps it could help me understand why my gut grew uneasy as Christmas approached, why Valentine's Day irritated the hell out of me, why Mother's Day just made me mad, why I was indifferent to Easter, why I wanted to hide as my birthday loomed on my calendar's horizon. Perhaps I'd find out why I wanted all my days to be ordinary, days that didn't call for any rituals, days I could fill at will, days I could spend using my own wits and imaginings.

My parents are both dead now. My mother outlived my father by twenty-five years, long enough for her to build a new life on her own, find a new relationship, and be a wife again for the last ten years of her life. During the decades that separated my parents' deaths, I started to feel my emotions differently—with my head as much as my body, as if I were pressing away the wrinkles with my cerebral steam iron.

My mother's death was the beginning of what I now think of as my "firestorm" phase. In her last years, my mother started telling me—only on the phone, not in person—that she loved me. The first time she did this, it unnerved me. It was not like my mother to say that. Love for each other was something we assumed, not something we said out loud.

When she said it again the next time we talked, and again the time after that, I realized that Mom had developed an undeniable need to say those words out loud. After a lifetime of not saying them, she was now determined to make certain I knew how she felt about me. For a few years, it became a welcome end to our conversations. "Well," she'd say, just before hanging up, "I do love you, you know." Feeling simultaneously uncomfortable and warmed, I responded the way she needed me to respond: "I love you too, Mom."

And then she lost the ability to talk on the phone. And then she lost the ability to talk at all. At many points in my life, I'd deliberately put distance between us. We'd been oil and water, she and me. Sometimes we mixed well together, enjoyed extended periods of compatibility, if not intimacy. Far too often, we didn't mix at all. When that happened, our polar differences solidified, like olive oil stored in the refrigerator.

And then she wasn't there any more. As soon as she was gone from this earth, I felt an overwhelming need for more of her. I had to find her again. But how do you find someone after they're gone for good? That's where viscerality comes in handy. My viscerality took me on a trek into the years my mother and I spent on this planet, both together and apart.

Twenty-Eight
Magnificent Mexican Sunsets

A winter holiday somewhere warm is a magnetic prize for many Canadians. We are attracted to tropical travel like filings to iron. Winter is wearing. It weighs on us, as if we carry it around on our bodies, an additional layer atop our puffy jackets, knit caps, thick mufflers, and furry boots. We seek relief from our darkest season in the brilliant warmth of the southern sun. We also look to escape our regular cycles of labour and life management, our successful highs and emotional lows. We don't pack those in our luggage. We especially don't pack worries about our mother's continuing loss of vocabulary, or her sudden inability to remember how to mix salad ingredients together in a bowl. We do our best to leave those things at home.

On the shores of Mexico's Banderas Bay, north of Puerto Vallarta and just beyond the resort town of Nuevo Vallarta, is Bucerias, a place many people see only when they pass through it on their way to somewhere else. A tight teeming town, Bucerias is where visitors and locals shop, eat, bargain, and beach together. A few years ago, I had the good fortune to visit Bucerias for a full glorious month.

Drawn to the shores of Banderas Bay by images of its sparkling water, I wanted the ocean's soothing rhythms to lull me to sleep every night. I'd been to Mexico a few times before, always on much shorter trips, always as a rushed tourist. For this trip, I had different goals. This time I wanted to settle in and get to know my chosen destination. I wanted to practice my mediocre Spanish. I wanted to write one poem every day, so that I'd return home with twenty-eight poems about picture-perfect Mexican sunsets in my notebook. For this trip, I wanted no emotional peaks. I wanted to feel nothing but peace and tranquility.

After a long travel day, my husband, daughter and I stood on the balcony of our rented third-floor condominium, as thirsty for the dazzling seascape in front of us as we were for the frothy ice-cold *cervezas* in our hands. The setting sun blazed the whole scene orange. As it vanished into the sea, we watched for the fickle flare of the green flash, the fleeting strobe that appears and disappears almost instantaneously, a phenomenon resulting from light refractions seen through the earth's dense atmosphere. Some people claim the green flash is a hallucination—that it doesn't exist. Some say it is visible only with an unobstructed view of the horizon at sea level. Others argue that it has been seen from the moon. That night, the sun disappeared without a hint of green, but I knew I wanted to see that flash. I had a feeling I'd need more than a little patience.

When we went to bed a few hours later, I left the balcony door to our bedroom wide open. Beside me, my husband fell asleep immediately. I read for a while, waiting for the waves to lull me to my slumber. I'd never slept so close to the ocean before. To my surprise, the surf sounds were not soft. The wind was calm that night, yet the incoming rollers made an aggressive roar, much stronger than I'd expected. But I'd come here to be lulled to sleep, and was determined it would happen. I lay awake much of that night waiting.

By lunchtime the next day, I was lounging on a chaise by the pool, my brand-new notebook in hand, ready to spend the afternoon writing my first poem. Located between our condo building and the water, the pool was elevated several feet above a wide expanse of beach. Anyone lounging beside the pool had a clear view down the long sandy curve that stretched in both directions along the bay. I settled in to watch all beach activity, looking for poetic inspiration. Half an hour later I'd managed to scrawl a few lines, but I was soon distracted by fragments of conversations from the people around me. I realized that I was in the company of familiar strangers. Almost everyone was from Canada. I found myself writing their words down on my page.

That guy selling silver jewellery must be hot in those long pants.
Why don't they wear sunglasses?
I heard that Mexicans cover up to keep their skin from getting any darker.
Am I brown yet?

I forced my mind back to my poem fragment and noticed that I'd used the word "glow" three times in three lines. I looked up at the sky in search of "glow" synonyms and saw huge black birds gliding above me. My daughter, a well-travelled conservation biologist who happens to know a lot about birds, lay on the chaise beside me. I asked her what they were. She opened one eye: *Magnificent frigatebirds, Mom.* What a great name, I thought as I repeated it to myself and jotted it down. As I looked at those two words, I was intrigued that we, the species with the power to name, the magnificent human race, had bestowed that word on a mere bird. But what a bird it was.

I couldn't stop watching the sky. They were everywhere. Their dark wings spanned seven feet from tip to tip, their silhouettes in the sky punctuated by long forked tails. By contrast, their bodies were puny, their physiques out of proportion, a grandiose design pushed to the max. Viewed from where I lay, they looked like flying Batman insignias, each one an ebony *W* slashed against the sky.

Gathering clouds hid the setting sun that evening, so I started a poem about what that day's sunset might have looked like. That night, again I waited for the pounding surf to lull me to sleep. After an hour, I closed the patio door to soften the noise, but I could still hear it through the glass. I spent yet another night with little sleep and no lulling.

The next morning, I stood on our balcony watching a local *vendedora* begin her day's work of selling merchandise along the beach. *Hola amigas*, she shouted to a group walking the sand. I listened carefully. *Mira! Abrigos de la playa! Compra!*

None of her potential customers looked at the colourful fabric beach wraps featuring butterflies or seahorses that covered her arms from shoulder to wrist. None of them showed any interest in the heavy backpack, bulging with more items for sale, strapped to her shoulders. When they had all passed by, the *vendedora* turned to watch them go. Then she stopped to let the waves wash over her feet. A big one tumbled in and foamed up past her knees. As the water receded, one flip-flop escaped her toes. With her heavy load, she couldn't bend over to retrieve it. As it floated away, a bikini-clad woman scampered to the rescue. She returned the sandal, but declined to purchase a butterfly sarong, was not even tempted by one with sequins on it. The *vendedora* shrugged and moved on to find other potential customers, eventually disappearing from my view.

That afternoon, I went for a walk along the beach. Above me, those big black birds again filled the sky. I knew more about them now. Their huge wings allow them to soar high above temperate ocean waters. They use warm air pockets to rise into the endless blue, where they carve smooth elegant arcs, so smooth that their wings don't seem to move at all. Their heads constantly turn, their eyes fixed on what's happening below. When something catches their attention, they descend, taking direct aim at their targets.

Unlike the ubiquitous brown pelicans or the blue-footed boobies they share the skies with—both species that hurl themselves into the waves to reach their prey—magnificent frigatebirds never, or at least only rarely, touch the water. Instead, they use their long beaks to pluck at food swimming just below the surface. Sometimes they dispense with the nuisance of fishing and wrest their meals from another bird's bill. Given the opportunity, they will even pull an almost-swallowed fish out of an unwary gullet. As I learned more about them, I realized that the magnificent frigatebird was a bit of a bully.

With evening approaching, I moved up to my balcony to wait for the sunset. I passed time watching a group of boogie boarders jockeying on white-capped waves, waiting for the best ride. Absorbed in their activity, I forgot about the setting sun. When I looked up it was gone, so I scribbled a few lines about the brilliant colours a completed sunset produces in the sky it left behind. I had no inclination to write a poem about boogie boarders, so I joined my family for happy hour.

That night, the waves hitting the beach were high. I closed the patio door, sat on the bed, and wrote in my notebook: *The ocean is loud. It pounds. Relentlessly. It cannot lull.* Then I inserted big orange plugs into my ears and slept through the night for the first time since our arrival.

For the next few days, my poetry efforts were disrupted by the very thing that draws so many shivering Canadians to Mexico in the winter: the weather. When the weather co-operates, days on Banderas Bay have a hypnotic rhythm. One runs into another. Is it Tuesday or Thursday? Yesterday or tomorrow? Does it even matter what day it is? When the weather changes, the rhythm changes too.

Our weather took a miserable turn that week. For a few days, we had no pink sunrises, no blue skies, no walks on the beach, no chance of a green flash sighting. Deluge followed deluge. No sunset poems could possibly come out of my brain in these conditions.

On the second straight day of rain, I joined a long-faced assemblage in the lobby of our condo building. We stared out at the puddles around the pool and up at the ominous grey sky. The friendly concierge shrugged his shoulders. *It never rains aquí en febrero, amigos.* We grumbled amongst ourselves. *This was not in the brochure.*

That night a huge wind blasted across the bay. A tropical depression birthed *una tormenta* that battered windows and doors, left cafés without roofs, felled trees across boulevards, sent umbrellas on frenetic flights through the air. As my husband struggled to secure the patio doors against the storm, I succumbed to that most primitive of human emotions, the one we inherited from our earliest ancestors, the one we most need to survive. Fear.

In that moment, I did what no mother should ever do: I hid behind my brave daughter. She assessed the situation, and in her calmest, most reassuring voice, suggested that we should put something on our bare feet in case the big patio windows shattered, and we had to evacuate. I ran to find my shoes and returned to be close to my daughter while my trembling hands struggled to tie my laces. By this time, my husband had managed to get the patio doors locked, was back in bed, and looked like he was already asleep. My daughter and I sat on the sofa, waiting, listening, ready to flee. After a while, she also went to bed. Eventually, I realized that our condo windows would hold, and I began to breathe easier. Still, long after the storm had abated, I sat on that sofa, unwilling to take my shoes off my feet. When I finally did remove them, even earplugs couldn't help me sleep.

The next morning, people all along Banderas Bay slowly emerged into the day, looking warily at the still-grey sky as they searched for deck chairs and umbrellas missing from their patios and balconies. Many found what they were looking for at the bottom of a swimming pool. In Bucerias, fallen branches littered the ground. Downed trees and power lines clogged the streets. Near our building, a caved-in brick wall made a whole block of sidewalk impassable. Broken sombrero kiosks lay toppled on their sides. If this was the work of a mere tropical depression, I never wanted to be anywhere near a full-blown hurricane.

Twenty-four hours later, the sun returned. Beach walkers came back to stride along the long curved expanse of sand again. Residents in our building began to smile once more and returned to their spots beside the pool. I reclaimed my regular lounge chair, pen in hand, my notebook opened to a fresh page.

The sky remained a brilliant cerulean blue all day, then shifted through a prism of colour as the sun began its descent. I more than watched it. I studied it, determined to create a good sunset poem that day. Each hour I eked out a few lines. Then I found myself jotting down snippets of a nearby poolside conversation I couldn't help overhearing.

> *Feel better today?*
> *Yup. But I had to wait for two hours at the local*
> *health clinic.*
> *They're all on mañana time here.*

I was surprised that the Mexican doctor spoke real
good English.
Did he help you?
He gave me a prescription and said I shouldn't
drink alcohol any more.
Like that's gonna happen.

When they jumped into the pool for their last dip of the day, I turned back to my unfinished verse, moved some words around and added more. Then I read over my work. The poem was a clunky mess, so I scratched it out. I found myself more interested in the dialogue I'd stolen, and wondered if I was better at eavesdropping than writing poetry. As the sun neared the horizon, I watched the sky, but no new poetic words sprang into my head, no green flash ignited my imagination.

The following days ran together. The sky stayed blue, never without birds to watch, especially those huge black floaters. I learned that magnificent frigatebirds don't like to touch down on water because they can't take off from water. Their splendid wings struggle on the rolling waves and their tiny unwebbed feet offer no propulsion assistance. Thus, they spend most of their lives in the air. Because their bodies are so light in comparison to their wings' capacity, they can stay aloft for up to a week and fly over two hundred kilometres without a rest. I watched a big male soar by at the same level as my balcony, and wondered how far it had flown to get to Bucerias. How does the mileage wear on them as the years pass? And as lightweight as they are, do they sometimes feel too heavy to soar?

One afternoon, I had just settled beside the pool when a piercing scream from out in the bay brought all movement to a halt. Beach walkers craned their necks, and everyone beside the pool stood up to see what was happening. We soon found the source of the cries, a dark spot out somewhere in the waves. The scream came again, but we couldn't tell whether it was a cry for help or a yelp of joy, its tenor somewhere between terror and rapture. No one moved for several minutes. The screaming continued, the dark shape now visible as a bobbing human head. Every few seconds an arm punched the sky. The concierge strolled out to have a look. *He's okay. No hay problema*, he said, smiling and motioning us all to return to our lounge chairs. Someone else commented that the continuing screams were a good sign. *If he really needed help, he would have disappeared by now*. Is that what we have to do to get help, I wondered. Disappear?

At this point, we were halfway through our Mexican sojourn. In my notebook, I had three incomplete sunset poems, and I didn't like any of them enough to finish them. I'd spent more time watching the area's winged wildlife than writing in my notebook.

My pen paused again when I noticed a flock of pelicans touching down on the water right in front of our building. Soon a feeding frenzy broke out. I watched those unwieldy big brown birds skim along the tops of the waves, rising up for brief mini-flights to gather momentum before plunging themselves into the briny bay. Seconds later they surfaced, always with a catch in their gullets. Accompanied by the squawking scavenger gulls that follow their talented friends to all the good fishing spots, the pelican horde lined up almost feather-to-feather on one long wave.

By now the situation was clear: I was turning into an accidental bird-watcher. I noticed birds everywhere I looked. In the sky. On the water. On the beach. I watched an elegant snowy egret prance across the sand on brilliant yellow legs that deftly avoided even the biggest rollers. Nearby, a little sandpiper scurried along, seeking a lunch of small crustaceans, or the innards of a seashell cast up by the incessant surf. Pure skinny energy, this little guy was a picture of confidence, unafraid of the human traffic around him, unperturbed by the pelicans and gulls noisily fishing out on the waves, unimpressed by the magnificent frigatebirds floating above.

Again I forced my attentions back to my poems, willed myself to think of different words for sun and awe. I couldn't. I'd run out of ways to describe a sinking orange orb. Magnificent as it was, the setting sun was beginning to bore me. And no matter how intently I watched it go down, I had yet to see the green flash.

Some mornings, I was up early, about an hour before sunrise. After watching the sky turn pink and then yellow and then a soft blue indicating the sun's arrival, I often decided on an early morning walk around town. On the way out of my building, I usually stopped to talk to the ever-present concierge. I spoke in Spanish. He responded in English. I tried Spanish again. He responded in English again. One day, I glanced down at what he was reading: an English language textbook. I should have thought of it myself, but he was the one who, at long last, made the obvious suggestion: if I helped him with his English, he would help me with my Spanish. I smiled. *Claro sí*, I said, with far too much pride. He smiled back as he answered: *Of course, señora.*

All was quiet on the streets when I started my walks, but soon coffee-seekers and joggers moved among the bicycles, jeeps, taxis, and water trucks. An hour later, I'd stop in for my exercise reward, a morning latte from the little café across the street from our building. The proprietor, a beautiful Mexican woman with flawless skin, waited patiently as I carefully placed my order in Spanish: *Buenos días, señora. Como estas? Yo necesito un latte decaf esta mañana.* Her response always came in

English: *did I want skim or whole milk?* And I always replied the same way: *Con leche skim, por favor.* It was a game we'd played ever since I arrived. Each day, I added at least one new Spanish word to my sentence. By this time, I was up to *con leche skim, por favor. Que lindo día es hoy!* As usual, her response came with a polite smile: *As you wish, señora.* Coffee in hand, I'd saunter back to my building.

One morning at the end of our third week, I saw a group of familiar faces standing in the foyer. My poolside acquaintances were waiting for their taxi, piles of luggage scattered at their feet. I stopped to wish them a good trip back to Canada, and lingered as they bid *adiós* to the concierge. They were still talking about that streak of bad weather we'd all endured. And the concierge was still trying to convince them that it had been unusual, that if they returned, it wouldn't happen again.

> *Yes. We know. It never rains here "en feb-ray-ro,*
> *amee-go."*
> *I hardly turned brown at all. No one will even know*
> *I was away.*
> *I've got a three-hour layover. That's what irks me.*
> *You'd think they'd want to make it more convenient*
> *for us to get here and back.*
> *Remember not to tip the cabbie.*

I watched them climb into their taxi, and waved goodbye. I was sad for them, but happy for me. I still had a week before I returned to my regular life. That evening, I sat on my balcony, trying not to blink as I studied the setting sun. *Please flash. Please flash.* And there it was. A flicker of intense lime-ish, yellow-ish, blue-ish green. But immediately gone. Had I seen it? Was it real or merely a wish fulfilled? I couldn't be sure.

For the remainder of my time in Bucerias, I watched in vain for another green flash. Every day, I jotted more words down in my notebook. Every day, the concierge and I had a brief chat. I'd ask him a question. *Cuantos niños tienes?* He'd answer immediately. *I have three children, señora.* I tried to answer equally as fast. *Me too. I mean, tres! Yo también.* His polite smile told me that I wasn't being very helpful to him. I needed better questions. I'd tried, unsuccessfully, to figure out how to ask about the scientific phenomenon known as the green flash in Spanish. I should have asked him to help me, but I didn't.

On each of my remaining days, after chatting to the concierge, I went for my morning walk and ordered my latte from the beautiful Mexican barista. And on each of my remaining days, she asked me in English if I wanted skim or whole milk. By now, I'd realized that she could only spend so much time with each customer, so my response was simply *skim, gracias.*

In the afternoons, I lay on my chaise counting down the days as I watched the magnificent frigatebirds fly over their pelican friends, always ready to take advantage of a good thieving opportunity. After a month of observing these striking birds, my sense was that their very magnificence was also their greatest flaw.

On departure day, I reflected back on the last four weeks, on the things I wouldn't pack in my luggage, but would take home with me nonetheless. In the mirror, I saw that my skin had a definite golden hue. In my voice, I heard that my Spanish was somewhat better than it had been a month ago, but I was still far from fluent. In both my head and my camera, I carried images of the townspeople diligently rebuilding their homes and businesses after *la tormenta*, an event now firmly established in the Bucerias trove of local lore. And my mind's eye held onto that one brilliant green flash, although I still wasn't certain whether or not I'd actually seen it.

As I packed my carry-on bag, I flipped through my half-filled notebook and saw that I'd written many words, phrases, and fragments, but not one complete sunset poem. Its remaining blank pages waited for me to forget about sunset poems, and think instead about how we spend so much time seeking out magnificence, sometimes not knowing it when we see it, or missing it when we're looking the other way.

Those Pesky Natal Days

The human ritual of marking individual birthdays started with the advent of the calendar, when people began to track time according to the sky, to notice when it got dark, when it got light, when the moon appeared, and when it didn't. Picture the first person who looked upwards and decided that the sky's patterns could give shape to our lives. I don't mean a physical picture of face, height, and hair colour. I mean a picture of that combination of curiosity and creativity, those upturned eyes, those hands that etched petroglyphs onto boulders with shards of granite, leaving behind timeless images of stick people living their lives.

In biblical times, the only people who could afford to have birthday parties were the nobility or other high-rankers. The elite classes put on lavish feasts for their entire courts. Everyone else watched. Sometimes they lined up along rivers to see elaborate barges drift by, or marched into the mountains of Galilee to witness a hillside extravaganza. I doubt they received loot bags filled with trinkets and candy.

Our contemporary birthday customs come from a variety of sources. We can thank the Greeks or the Germans—depending on which internet resource you believe—for that most palatable of birthday traditions, the cake. The candles came later and symbolize life or light or the moon—again depending on your preferred resource. Apparently the custom of sending birthday cards began in Britain when people dispatched birthday greetings to those they were unable to see in person. Today, we no longer have to send a physical card. They're in danger of being totally replaced by e-mails, Twitter feeds, and Facebook postings.

Birthdays are such common celebrations that it's difficult to imagine they haven't always been a happiness-on-demand day. Wary of the birthday party idea, early Christians believed that people were susceptible to evil spirits on those days, and viewed birthday festivities as pagan rituals that should be abandoned. Even today, some very orthodox believers still view overt birthday celebrations as something God would disapprove of. How anyone can claim to know what God disapproves of is beyond me. I mean no religious disrespect when I say that citing the bible as evidence of God's interior thoughts and expectations isn't proof of anything. The word of God, written by whom? For what purpose?

I imagine a brown-robed monk, elevated in the eyes of his community not only by his attire, but also by his unusual ability to read and write. Very few people had those skills back then, almost none of them women. My imaginary monk sits down on a hard bench and pulls a piece of parchment towards his body. Quill in hand, small jar of inky liquid at the ready, he begins to record heavenly words. But what words? How do they come into his head and what assumptions do they carry with them? It's entirely possible that my monk wasn't on the receiving end of divine communication. At least some of those biblical words are his own and imbued with what was happening in his life that day. Maybe the village had just experienced an epidemic. Maybe the crops were dying in the fields. Maybe no one ever wished him a happy birthday.

I wish I could remember my first one, my zero birthday, the day I squeezed out between my nineteen-year-old mother's legs, pushed out of her warm womb by powerful contractions into a hospital room of glaring fluorescent lights and eyes peering out from masked faces.

What did I feel? What does any infant feel at the moment of birth? I doubt that it's joy or love. More likely, a combination of distress emotions. Fear about this strange, harsh new world. And probably anger at being disturbed, at being so rudely ejected from a place of comfort.

And what's the first thing we need after our arrival? Soothing. We need something to settle us down, something to suck on that will ease that fear and anger, something to bring us contentment, something to allow our infant psyches to embrace the possibilities of joys ahead, something to prepare us for the inevitable sorrows. It's possible that from the moment of our birth, we spend the rest of our lives looking for pacifiers, those soothing elements, healthy and unhealthy, anything to calm our first-felt emotions. At birth, we are all addicts in the making.

Our early birthday narratives are an intimate family construction of fact, memory, and imagination. On one of my birthdays, maybe my thirteenth or fourteenth, I asked my mother how she felt when I was born, a loaded moody-teenager question designed to get my mother to tell me how thrilled she was to have beautiful little me come into her life. She didn't answer, just looked as if I'd asked her why her heart pumped blood to her hands and feet. Then she went back to preparing a chicken for the barbecue or chopping onions for spaghetti sauce.

If I remember correctly, I persisted and asked my question again. And I think she resisted answering again. My reconstruction of what followed is undoubtedly flawed, but it probably went something like this. I changed my question and asked what time of day I was born. Mom thought for several minutes before saying she thought it was just after suppertime. I felt a little hurt that the answer wasn't immediately in her head. How could she not carry the moment of my birth with her every minute of every day? Too caught up in my adolescent anxieties, I didn't consider that she'd been a mother for a long time by then, almost a third of her life. With four children (and one more yet to come), our various births must have blurred together in her head. Or not. Like most women in the 1950s, she was under a general anaesthetic for all her childbirths. Maybe she really didn't remember.

Even at that, I probably wasn't finished with my questions. What was my crib like? What colour was my favourite blanket? And my mother probably answered each one with another question. Why did I want to know? What did it matter? The only firm details I can attest to are these. The summer of my zero birthday had been a hot one. Daily temperatures and humidity levels remained high. Day after sticky, sunny day dragged by between my expected arrival date and my eventual entrance. Mom's strongest memory of the day I was born seemed to be that I'd kept her waiting much too long in that heat.

That's all I know of that long-past August day in Winnipeg. All we know about our zero birthdays, and the first two or three or four that follow, comes from old pictures, from what other people tell us, from the nuggets in their memories—that is, the ones they decide to share, their choices shaped by how they want us to think about that day. Or, as in my mother's case, how she didn't want me to think about it at all.

Mine is a summer birthday. It usually falls on or near that no-name holiday at the beginning of August—the holiday

Monday that's a holiday for no reason except that it's summer in Canada—a day I've always associated with backyard barbecues or swimming in Lake Winnipeg. Both are memories born from nostalgia. The number of times I've actually immersed myself in a lake on my birthday are probably fewer than my memory bank wishes were so.

My parents gave me a little Brownie camera for my tenth or eleventh birthday. My best friend got the same camera from her parents on her birthday that same year. Soon afterwards, we stood with our exotic new gadgets in our hands, those mystical things that somehow captured images of anything we pointed them at. What would happen, we wondered, our eyes growing bigger, if we pointed them at each other and snapped two pictures at the very same moment? Would the picture-making waves cancel each other out when they collided? Would there be a puff of smoke?

We stood back-to-back, duel-style, and counted off five steps away from each other. Then we turned and raised our cameras to our eyes. On the count of three, two simultaneous clicks sounded as one. That was it. Nothing else happened. We shrugged, laughed, and ran off to the beach. When we got our developed films back, I had a picture of her taking a picture of me, and she had a picture of me taking a picture of her. We compared the two shots. Except for the hair colour (she was a brunette, I was blonde), the images were almost identical. We even had the same stance, right hip thrust out to the side, left knee bent.

I'm convinced that my teenaged hip-thrusting stance is a classic Leo pose. I don't have much faith in astrology, but I'm well aware that I fall under the sign of Leo. That means that when I'm pontificating about something that impassions me, such as how difficult it is for a left-hander to live in a right-handed culture, I expect people to listen. I've studied Leos.

And, as a Leo, I expect that I've been studied too. Which is fine. We are okay with being gazed upon. This is because we Leos are often our own suns. We're ambitious and enthusiastic. We demand to be noticed. We especially want to be noticed more than other Leos. But there's a downside to all this brightness. We can also be arrogant, condescending, and overly dramatic. One thing we aren't is uncaring.

I admit to having demonstrated all the above leonine characteristics at various times in my life. A few years ago, I started to get heat rashes on my skin during hot weather: deep, itchy, blistery, ugly rashes. My doctor told me that I had developed an allergy to the sun. Nonsense, I replied. I can't be allergic to the sun. I'm a Leo.

I grew up in a household where four out of the seven occupants were Leos. Just imagine the screaming silences and the silent screamings. Just imagine the performances, the soliloquies, the entrances and exits. No wonder my father, one of the non-Leos, spent so much time telling his Leo-laden pride not to be so sensitive. No wonder my mother, one of the Leos, spent so much time clenching her teeth.

I enjoy other people's birthdays. I like buying the cards and presents, putting candles on birthday cakes. I don't like the song at all. For a short little ditty with a copyright supposedly worth five million dollars, the Happy Birthday song is simply not very good. It's grating and trivial. The lyrics consist of only five provided words, with a blank space for the sixth that singers have to fill in themselves. The sentiment is a tedious repetitive demand to be happy. Most often sung at a lethargic, dirge-like pace, the words come out like cooling taffy. This causes the melody's forward momentum to be even slower than molasses in January. I know that's a cliché, but if you've ever tried to spoon molasses out of a jar that's been stored in a cold cupboard, you'll know how accurate it is. Once started at that January-molasses pace, the Happy Birthday song plods along and is almost impossible to speed up. Sometimes I deliberately start singing it fast, in brisk allegro-style, an effort that usually causes confusion because I get all the way to the end before others have finished the second line.

I enjoy planning informal birthday celebrations for other people, not big parties, just dinner. An ingredient will inspire the menu, a savoury ingredient, like rosemary or spinach, something the celebrant favours. When my children were small, I held birthday parties for them every year, usually in the basement of our house. During the week before, I would spend a few days gathering what I needed—hot dogs, buns, cake, candles, balloons, and take-home loot bags that I filled with trinkets from K-Mart. And a present, usually something practical like a winter jacket or new snowboots. Conveniently, my children all have fall birthdays, so I bought them what they needed to keep warm during the upcoming winter. The age of the birthday child determined the number of people who would attend the party. When I filled out the invitations, I always indicated, in bold print and underlined, exactly what time the parents should drop their children off, and exactly what time they should arrive to pick them up. These parties never lasted more than two hours. One year, when our twins were eight or nine, I got a migraine just before the guests arrived. I had no choice but to lie down in a dark, quiet room, leaving my husband to run the party. That was good planning on my part.

The birthday parties I used to stage would not suffice these days. Things have changed. Today, children's parties must have a theme. It might be a superhero party with red capes for all, or a princess party with mandatory tiaras, or a pirate party with a big prize for the best eye patch. Everything at the party has to be connected to the theme, especially the cake, which ideally will have more than one tier. My old rectangular slab cake would not do.

The decorations—balloons are no longer adequate on their own—must reinforce the theme. The napkins must go with the cups must go with the tablecloth must go with the loot bags. A hand-painted drawing displayed on an easel by the entrance is an effective touch. That way, all guests will pick up on the theme immediately. Walking into a room painted pink with feather boas and sequin-encrusted ballet slippers hanging from the ceiling leaves no room for doubt.

Of course, the food must connect to the theme. It should also be homemade, organic, and non-allergenic. Also required is a gourmet appetizer table—perhaps a selection of tapenades and artisan cheeses—to feed the guests' parents, who no longer drop off and pick up their children. They come for the whole thing, and must be entertained too. My kids are lucky they grew up before this trend took hold. I'm very impressed by theme parties, but relieved that I don't have to throw one.

Yes, I like other people's birthdays, but I don't like my own birthday one little bit. One day in late May or early June, the dreaded thought tiptoes into my head. My birthday is coming. Crap, my birthday is coming. When this happens, my esophagus constricts immediately. Not because I'm another year older. I'm quite reconciled to that. Even if I weren't, what could I do about it? The moving sidewalk of life is never closed for repair.

To distract myself after that initial birthday thought wanders in, I start thinking about how I want to spend my day. My first idea is always the same: I just want to disappear. No obligations, no hanging around to receive birthday wishes, no smiling when I really feel like roaring into the wind.

I don't like opening birthday presents, especially in front of the people who have given them to me, who sit in my line of vision smiling with eager anticipation. In *The Gift of Thanks*, Margaret Visser writes about a Japanese custom that discourages gift-givers from watching gift-receivers open their presents. It's poor etiquette. Instead, givers leave their parcels without fanfare and receivers open them later, released from the pressure of a proper response. I think I would like that. When I open gifts in front of a large group of people, what falls into my hands is secondary, because I'm hoping that my smile is big enough, that I'm not over-reacting or under-rewarding my donor, that I'm appropriately grateful without resorting to an "I've always wanted one of these" gusher statement. I wince when I recall times I have gushed.

I don't mind the candles. In fact, I like the blowing part. I have good lungs, and almost always get every flame out with one gust. But then again, I haven't actually had candles to blow out for a number of years now. Once the number gets high, the motivation to put candles on a cake declines.

Sometimes I tell my family not to do anything for my birthday. This is a dangerous instruction, and they know it. If they take me at my word, I'm disappointed. I know, and they have come to know, that I will sulk if the day approaches and I sense nothing special is in the works. When they sense what I'm sensing, they throw a gathering together. My next move is a feeble attempt to back out of whatever they've come up with. It's a nasty circle. I know what I'm doing, and yet can't stop myself.

For significant birthdays, the ones ending in five or zero, especially the ones ending in zero, the throat constrictions and pit-throbbing in my stomach are much worse. Several times, I decided to deal with these intense birthdays by surrounding myself with my extended family for a weekend of merriment and cooking, cakes and cleanup, conversations and cameras. In the photos, I am smiling and happy, but when I look at them, I remember feeling that I just wanted everything to be over. The frenzy exhausted me. Surrounded by people I love, I looked forward to the moment they all left. Not until recently, when I uncloseted myself as an introvert who has spent most of her life masquerading as an extrovert, did I understand those feelings. A birthday is a strong demand from our closest allies to be happy. They want us to be happy, at least most of them. And if we aren't, they are disturbed, disappointed, anxious. But happy can be hard work.

Several years ago, my husband gave me a guitar for one of those significant birthdays, one ending in a zero. I was opening gifts and cards in a room full of family. Finally, I came to the card from him. I don't remember what the card looked like, just the words inside: "Look downstairs in the closet." When I returned with my present in my hands, I may have gushed a little.

For a long time, I'd been telling him that I wanted to learn how to play a guitar, but I never thought he'd go out and buy me one. I was excited to hold it, but didn't quite know how. It felt awkward. That weekend, one of my sisters showed me how to play a few chords. During the next few weeks, I picked it up each day and strummed my fingers across its strings. One day, I tried strumming with a pick for the first time and immediately dropped it into the hole in the middle of the guitar. It took me half an hour to shake it out. A few times, I even turned the pages of the *How to Play the Guitar* book my husband had tucked into the case. He'd bought a travel case for it, too, one with straps on it like a backpack. I had a fleeting image of myself walking through an airport, wearing it over my lime-green trench coat.

But soon I stopped touching my guitar. I kept it in sight, safe in its case, leaning in a corner of our television room. My husband, to his credit, never asked me about it out loud. But the questions I saw in his eyes hung in the air. What's up? You said you wanted one. Why aren't you playing it?

The truth is that it scared me. After so many years of stating this unexamined desire, I backed away from it. What if I failed? What if I couldn't do it? What if my hands were too small to manage the contortions required to fret chords? And why bother? At this point in my life, what was the point? I wasn't going to play in public. I wasn't about to become a musician. I wasn't looking to post videos of me playing and singing "If You Could Read My Mind" on YouTube.

My guitar went unplayed for more than three years. Then, a year after my mother's death, I picked it up and started plunking away one afternoon when I was home alone. When no other ears but mine were within hearing distance, I went to it each day and taught myself the notes. And then some chords. And then some progressions. My fingers hurt. In the beginning, my index finger got to the point of bleeding. Soon I had guitar calluses on my fretting fingers, and felt pleased. Just getting the calluses was an accomplishment. I stuck with it, welded myself to my guitar for at least half an hour every day. After a few weeks, I could play a simple version of "Ode to Joy" and have it sound like "Ode to Joy."

And then I knew why I wanted it. For me. I wanted to play the guitar just for myself. Here, in what could be the November of my life, I've learned a new language to think in, one that exits through my fingers.

I'm happy to keep having birthdays because that means I'm still alive. However, the day itself is still uncomfortable for me. My best birthday in recent memory included no lake swimming, but it did feature a backyard barbecue. It was a relatively painless event. I spent most of it travelling, riding in the passenger seat as my husband steered us west from Jasper to the Okanagan Valley. The ride was smooth, the massive granite of Mount Robson clear against the sky, unobscured by the clouds it usually attracts.

Taking a long road trip on my birthday was a good idea. As I sat watching the British Columbia interior pass by my window, largely cut off from the outside world, I felt better. During the ride, I mulled over my birthday resistance once more, but I didn't come up with any new answers. That's okay. I'm resigned to dreading my birthday as it looms, resigned to not wanting any special attention—and expecting it anyway. I can't seem to fix this behaviour, which makes me wonder if it's genetic. Perhaps I inherited it from my mother. Like her, I consider myself a practical, pragmatic person, whose default position is to be upbeat about the days that make up my weeks and months. Yet every year, my approaching birthday almost derails me. I'm still not certain whether it's a fear of disappointment, a fear of disappointing others with my disappointment, or a simple wish that our social world didn't place so much emphasis on age.

What I do know is that the day after my birthday will be a good day. I will feel normal again, relieved, and somehow refreshed. For about ten months. I also know that when it's all over and I crawl into bed that night, I will feel somewhat sad and a little let down that I have to wait for a whole year before my natal day comes around again. Maybe that's my personal birthday party theme: smiles and tears, sad happiness and happy sadness. Maybe those two emotions are closer than we think.

Death by Dementia

It shouldn't surprise us. We know it's coming. We know in October when repeated hand-washings and standing in line for flu shots become common daily activities. I know in November when the rabbits in the park near my house turn from tawny brown to pure white. I feel sorry for them when our fickle weather tricks us with a brown December, leaving those rabbits hopping down the bare back alleys or across the dead grass, their white fur betraying them.

Over the years, my winter survival strategies have included puffy coats, thick fleece-lined boots, steaming mugs of gut-warming beverages, and belly-filling comfort food. The initial comfort of January's respite from the Christmas frenzy soon dissipates as it lapses into a lumbering series of short days and long nights. The first month's slow move through its sun-starved dark weeks eventually does result in more hours of daylight, but not necessarily more warmth. Thus, a recent addition to my winter survival strategy includes time in a warmer climate. Winter is for the young, and while I still feel young in many ways, I don't feel winter-young.

I grew up in Manitoba and have spent much of my adult life in Alberta. Both provinces are home to me. People who haven't lived in either one tend to define them by their winters. Their physical and seasonal boundaries are similar. Both are physically connected to the territories in the north and our boisterous neighbour to the south, but not to each other. Yet for me, Manitoba and Alberta are connected in my sense of self, with Manitoba winters ever so slightly edging out Alberta's in the harshness category. In Manitoba, winter could arrive before Halloween and might not depart until May. When I lived there, we hoped for, but did not expect, any respite between October and May. Like Manitoba, Alberta's winters also arrive in October and can overstay their welcome to May, but Albertans expect respites in between, mild days and weeks where we can catch our breath. When those respites don't show up, we feel deprived.

Weather dominates casual conversations in both provinces. I used to think this was a trite way for people to communicate without much effort or genuine interest in each other. In recent years, I've come to realize that weather is a much more complex topic. It connects us in ways that we feel under our skin and in our bones.

With fondness, if not nostalgia, I remember my Manitoba tobogganing days. Even in prairie-flat Winnipeg, we found hills steep enough to send our sleds racing to the bottom. Many tobogganers desired crash landings, sudden separations between their sleds and their bodies, limbs flailing from inside swirling white clouds. That was not for me. I preferred coasting to a calm finish, after which I'd stand at the bottom looking back towards the top. I liked measuring the distance with my eyes, noting how far along the flats I'd managed to coax my sled. Then I'd grab the rope and begin the trudge back up the hill again.

My toboggan was the usual wooden slat version, shaped like a candy cane, big enough for two. My friend down the street had an identical one. Heck, everyone in the neighbourhood had the same toboggan. Our parents all shopped at the local Canadian Tire store.

The nearest toboggan hill was several long blocks from where we lived. Sometimes, on a Saturday or Sunday afternoon, my mother would drive us there, the ends of our toboggans extending beyond the open trunk. If Mom couldn't drive us, we'd walk, our sliders trailing along behind on the snow-packed sidewalk. Frigid temperatures didn't deter us. Temperatures were numbers adults paid attention to. We liked the icy tingle on our cheeks and the feel of our eyelashes freezing together.

I haven't been on a toboggan in a very long time. It's an appealing thought in its simplicity. As the years pile up, life can no longer be simple because life experiences not only accumulate, they also complicate. And even though we deny them with emphatic statements like "If I had it to do all over again, I wouldn't change a thing," we have regrets, remnants that pester us, say "I wish I'd handled that situation differently, I wish I'd stifled my inappropriate laughter, I wish I'd paid attention to innocuous details, I wish I'd felt my viscerality more, let it move me, let it teach me." Yes, I wrote that whole last sentence in the first-person plural, preferring the company of "we" to the solitariness of "me," as I wondered why it took so many years for me to learn to listen to my gut.

As a child still living with my parents, I always assumed that my mother loved the month of December and all the Christmas activity as much as I did. She seemed to handle it all so well, the crazy crush of the morning present opening and cleanup, followed by a sit-down brunch and managing the afternoon food preparations, after which she'd see that we were all dressed in our good clothes. Finally, she'd settle her pearls around her neck, ready to greet my grandparents when they arrived for the traditional turkey dinner. Now I wonder if she might have preferred January, especially back in the days when all her children were still in her care. Not until I myself had for many years performed the duties of what I've come to think of as "The Christmas General"—the one who plans, shops, wraps, mails, decorates, stocks the house, and makes the goodies—did I realize the fatigue my mother must have felt as each Yuletide approached.

Perhaps, eventually, like the adult me, Mom saw how the Christmas decorations that sparkled so brightly as we unpacked them soon lost their lustre, how a tinselly tackiness came over them almost as soon as we'd finished hacking the Christmas turkey to bits. Perhaps, like me, she grew eager for the restored simplicity of our normal surroundings once the decorations were stowed away in the basement for another year. Perhaps, like me, she welcomed the end of December's frenzied holiday season, the relief from relentless festivity as the slower pace of January took over. Perhaps, like me, she savoured the simple clean taste of low-fat yogurt after the indulgence of her melt-in-the-mouth Christmas shortbread. She made the same recipe all her life, not even looking at the short list of ingredients written out on a yellowing index card, instructions not required. Then came the Christmas that she forgot the instructions she hadn't needed for more than half a century.

The visit to the doctor's office happened just after Easter. On a crisp but sunny spring day, I drove from Edmonton to Calgary. I felt uneasy as I climbed into my mother's car along with Mom and one of my sisters. My mother's husband drove us to the clinic, where we sat in silence in a waiting room, its walls painted a soft blue. The clinic's staff moved around without urgency, wearing warm smiles and street clothes. I wanted to be elsewhere. Anywhere but there.

Soon we were directed into an office. The geriatric specialist who greeted us was impossibly young. He wore a dark shirt, open at the neck. No tie. No white lab coat. His words came out slowly, with impeccable enunciation. As he spoke, he made eye contact, first with my mother and then, one by one, with the rest of us. His topic was Primary Progressive Aphasia, a somewhat rare form of dementia. It was the condition my mother had been diagnosed with a few months earlier.

We sat in a semi-circle in front of the young doctor's desk, my mother and her husband on the right, my sister and I on the left. I don't remember if anyone attempted any small talk. Mostly, we waited for the doctor to speak. He started with a question.

"Have you noticed any deterioration in your mother's language skills recently?" the doctor asked in the direction where my sister and I sat.

I answered. Of course, I answered. As the oldest of my mother's five children, it was my job to answer.

"Yes," I said. "For about two years now. She forgets words, can't find the ones she needs when she needs them. She can't complete her sentences. We have to prompt her."

My mother's head swivelled in my direction, her face contorted into a deep scowl. Her brown eyes had turned black and locked into mine until I pulled my gaze away and looked back at the doctor.

"Have you noticed any deterioration in your wife's language skills recently?" the doctor then asked my mother's husband of five years.

"No," he said. "I haven't noticed anything at all."

Beside him, my mother nodded vigorously and aimed her best, most radiant smile at the doctor.

For the rest of the appointment, the doctor focused most of his attention on my mother. Very gently, using her first name, he explained what was happening to her, and how her condition would affect her life. She sat quietly, nodding occasionally, smiling politely when he asked her a question. He gave her a lot to think about, but I don't remember her saying much in response. The doctor recommended another visit, very soon, as well as more tests and speech therapy. He strongly recommended counselling for the whole family. We all nodded and left.

As the four of us walked back to the car, I felt a knot in my gut. I wanted to be somewhere else. Anywhere else.

Two days later, back home in Edmonton, I sat on the stairs leading up to my bedroom, holding the phone to my ear with one hand and pulling at my hair with the other. My mother's voice was loud and hard. "Why are you doing this to me? Why can't you leave me alone?"

I took a calming breath to level my voice. "Mom, please don't ignore this. Please go back to that doctor. Please do the things he's asking you to do. Make plans for how you want to handle this now. Please, Mom."

"There's nothing wrong with me," she said. "This happens to everybody. That doctor is a quack."

Sometimes she had no trouble at all finding the words she needed.

It's a hole, this aphasia thing, a growing gap in the front temporal region of the brain. On the Mayo Clinic's website, the description of Primary Progressive Aphasia (PPA) consists of six sentences made up of one hundred and twenty words, eighteen of which are primary or progressive or aphasia. From those words, I learned that people afflicted with this condition have difficulty expressing thoughts and following conversations. They may eventually lose all language abilities. One sentence notes that the condition progresses slowly. When I read that, my first thought was that progress is a strange word to use—both in this description and in naming the condition. It should be regress, because there is no forward movement in PPA. There is only reversion, retrogression, decline, deterioration, degeneration. At the beginning, it's a slow subtle slide. Towards the end, it's freefall.

What's missing from the Mayo Clinic's description, and from all others I've found, is what actually happens as time passes. What these descriptions don't include is when to expect further deterioration, how long each phase will take, and how utterly devastating it will be to watch. And I know why these things are missing from those descriptions. They are too hard to write. The condition's progression forward is so regressive that spelling it out in detail would be unreadable for those who have to deal with it. Words are inadequate preparation for this process because once started, its inevitable movement is towards the ultimate regression.

More than three years passed. My mother continued to ignore her situation. She smiled a lot when words failed her, which gradually evolved into every time she tried to speak. She forgot how to make her Christmas shortbread. She forgot how to set a table or read the newspaper. She rarely referred to any of her children or grandchildren by name any longer. She didn't drive, didn't walk very far, didn't leave her condo much. Her physical presence changed as well. The smile she now used as her main form of communication was nervous and fleeting. Her once-strong body looked frail. Her once-youthful looking face had become gaunt and pallid. Her hair—Mom had always been fastidious about her hair—was neglected and lank. As a family, we were confused about what to do and weary, oh so weary, with worry. Finally, my mother's husband said that he couldn't manage her daily care at home any longer.

When I visited Mom at the assisted living residence she moved into, or rather was moved into by us—without her consent, at great emotional cost to all, but especially her—I usually found her in the dining room. I say "usually" with reservation, because I visited her at that location only four times. In a weak defense for that paltry number, I've learned to remind myself that she lived there for just four months, that I lived in a different city, and our harsh Alberta winter was harsher than usual that year. To compensate for my absence, I phoned her more often. That solution came to an end when Mom took the telephone we'd installed in her room and drowned it in her bathroom sink.

The first time I went to visit, it was December. While parking the car, I realized that I didn't have anything to give her, so I popped into a nearby drugstore and bought a glittery plastic snowman with a red scarf around its neck. She lit up when she saw it, as if its two AA batteries were connected to her, not the snowman. I was pleased when she put it on the nightstand beside her bed. Maybe she was adjusting to her new situation after all.

On my next visit, I found Mom sitting at the nurse's station, looking down at her hands. The nurse on duty seemed to be keeping an eye on her. I discovered later that sometime during the previous day, Mom had taken another resident's walker and hidden it in her room. My mother, who had never stolen anything in her life, was sitting at the nurse's station, on probation for bad behaviour. I don't know why she wanted the walker. At that point, she could still walk on her own.

On my next two visits, I found Mom sitting in the dining room, alone. Both times, she sat at a table, her back to the wall, looking out at the empty room, focusing on nothing. She just sat there. Eyes open, hands in her lap, not moving any muscle in her body. Both times, I watched her for a few moments before making my presence known, watched to see if I could find any hint of what she might be thinking about. As I looked at her, I tried to imagine my brain leaking words, tried to feel what it would be like to have the lake of my vocabulary draining a paragraph or two at a time through some unseen puncture in my head.

In between visits, I wrestled with questions. Unanswerable questions. How does one think without words? Is it even possible? Perhaps with an object, a common everyday object, I could see myself picturing a chair in my mind and showing someone else the shape of a chair with my hands, gesturing that I required a chair, even offering a chair for another to sit in. All without words. But what about something like fear? How does one deal with fear without words? How does one prevent a dreadful darkness from overwhelming a brain with a rapidly dwindling number of words available to help manage that fear? The questions themselves made me afraid.

On a cold dark March evening, when winter had not yet departed from Calgary, I walked into the long-term care facility Mom had been transferred to earlier that day. The assisted living residence had declared it could no longer manage her needs. In the last few weeks, Mom had started to lose the ability to feed herself and her walking had become unsteady.

The long-term care facility was in an area of Calgary I wasn't familiar with, and it took me a while to find it in the dark. Once there, I checked in at the front entrance. A friendly woman greeted me with warmth, the right amount of warmth, not too familiar, but welcoming enough to coax me in: "Yes, your mother arrived this afternoon. She's settling into her room. I'm sure she'll be pleased to see you."

I followed the instructions the friendly receptionist provided: left down the hall past the elevators, enter the code into the panel beside the doors to the secured wing, pass through those doors, pause to make certain they close behind you, walk through the dining room, turn right, and go halfway down the hall.

My mother's room was spacious and clinical. All the floor and furniture surfaces were hard and smooth, easy to clean. In the corner was a single hospital-style bed. Mom sat on the edge of it, her feet on the floor. She was wringing her hands when she looked up and saw me standing in the doorway.

"You," she said.

I sat down beside her and gave her a hug. She responded by getting up and walking across the room to a large cabinet. I noticed that her steps were slower and more deliberate than the last time I'd seen her. She opened the door to the cabinet and I saw her now-meagre wardrobe of clothes hanging neatly from the rod. She touched her blouses, one by one. I thought I could hear a gargling sound coming from her throat. Then she closed the door, walked back to the bed, and sat down beside me.

"Out," she said. "Out, out, out."

I knew she didn't mean that I should leave. I knew she meant that she wanted out. I did too.

On a dresser beside the wardrobe, I spied a black-and-white photograph of her parents, my long-dead grandparents. Knowing that the sight of old pictures like this had recently had a calming effect on her, I held it out towards her.

She pushed it away. "All dead," she said. "Dead."

I put my arm around her shoulders. She shrugged me off.

A minute or so later, she looked at me. Her eyes narrowed as she said, "You never do anything."

I kissed her goodnight and told her I'd be back in the morning. On my way out, I asked the nurse on duty to check in on her.

The next morning, I found Mom in the dining room. I sank down into the chair beside her and watched as she toyed with a piece of toast, her breakfast plate still in front of her. I picked up a spoon and fed her a small mouthful of scrambled egg. My mother had always preferred her eggs poached, but she accepted this morsel.

Across the table, another resident sat in a wheelchair. When this woman's gaze fell on me, I smiled and said good morning. She responded by saying "Goddammit, goddammit, goddammit!"

I saw my mother shake her head a little in the woman's direction. The gesture made me chuckle to myself, as I remembered how my much-younger mother used to shake her head at me when I'd done or said something she didn't like. My old mother looked away from the swearing woman and smiled at me. "You have a nice mom," she said. And we both laughed.

Two weeks later, it was still March and the roads were still snowy. Alberta was caught in a winter that seemed determined to last forever. Again I drove from Edmonton to Calgary, my two daughters with me this time. We found my mother in her room, lying on her bed. A wheelchair sat in the corner. A nurse told me that Mom could no longer walk on her own and had lost all ability to feed herself. We got her into the wheelchair and went to a private dining room, where we tried to get some lunch into her.

Before we left that day, I kissed her on the forehead and said, "I'm going to Arizona for a week, Mom. I'll come for a visit as soon as I get back." She didn't respond. On our way out, a nurse promised that she'd make sure my mother ate some supper that night.

For the return trip to Edmonton, I crawled into the back seat of my car and let my daughters drive me home. I didn't want to think. I lost myself in the sound of my daughters' voices as they chatted quietly to each other in the front. I stared out the window at my province's snow-streaked landscape. But all I could see was my mother's face.

I was away when Mom was admitted to hospital. The day after I'd arrived in Arizona, Mom had been found unresponsive in her room. While I'd enjoyed a leisurely walk to the local coffee shop for my morning latte, drinking in the deep blue Arizona sky, my mother had been taking the first ambulance ride of her life. When I received the news, I could picture where she was, lying on a high white bed in the same hospital where three of her grandchildren were born, the same one where my grandmother had died almost twenty years ago.

Over the next six days, regular updates from family members on the scene kept me apprised of her condition. I spent that April week with my cellphone always in hand, a preoccupied Canadian visitor warming herself among the Palo Verde and mesquite trees that fill Arizona's landscape, lush in their spring finery, their tiny yellow blossoms brilliant against the bluest of skies. I needed sunglasses just to look at those trees. Against their brilliance, my mind screened the image of a white or beige or pale green hospital room, my mother positioned squarely in its centre, an intravenous drip rehydrating her body, my siblings gathered around her, chatting with each other, handling the family crisis without me. "Don't come back just yet," they said. "She's coming out of it." A wary calm settled over me and I held onto it as if I were water-skiing behind a boat, gliding on smooth waters, knowing that the rope would inevitably escape my grasp.

On my last day in Arizona, I had a free afternoon before my flight home. I decided to take a guided tour through famed architect Frank Lloyd Wright's winter home and studio, Taliesin West. At first, I put my phone's ring on silent and shoved it into my pocket. But it felt heavy on my leg as I started to walk away, so I changed my mind. I unlocked the car and threw my phone into my luggage.

Built in 1937, Wright's sprawling estate consists of low-slung structures that blend in with the Sonoran desert, and feel as natural as the cholla, barrel, and saguaro cactuses that grow up the hillsides of the surrounding McDowell Mountain Range. During the two-hour oasis of that tour, I floated, let go of all links to my world, surrendered myself to a thirst for neutral information. Content in the anonymous solitude that comes from being in a group of strangers, I heard, but didn't listen to, the voice of our guide, took comfort from her constant presence, as if she were part of the warm desert backdrop.

Taliesin West isn't a museum locked in the past. It's a functioning school where architecture students learn, and visual artists produce new work. In the sculpture garden I lagged behind the group, lingered under the mid-afternoon sun, fascinated by the various bronze shapes perched atop cement pillars or planted into the stones of the patio. I found myself especially drawn to a small female figure encased almost entirely in a full-length hooded cape, her body completely covered except for her hands and face, her eyes fixed on some point beyond this earth. I took a picture of her, using my camera's lens to frame her billowing garment against the rough rock of Wright's walls.

After the tour finished, I drove from Taliesin West to Phoenix's Sky Harbor Airport. As I passed the many signs directing traffic through the maze of lanes into the airport area, I felt my usual urge to insert a Canadian "u" in the American version of "Harbor." The word looks unfinished without it, harsher somehow, not as safe as it should. Once I'd steered my way through the coiled ramps that form the entry to the airport's rental-car building, I returned my car and boarded the shuttle bus for the terminal. Only then did I pull out my phone. I saw five voice messages waiting for me—two from my husband, one from my daughter, two from my sister—and knew without listening to any of them that my mother was gone.

I was calm as I went through airport security and passed along the moving sidewalks to my plane's gate, calm as I boarded and watched the dusky lights of Phoenix fade behind us on our climb into the night. I didn't read a word on that flight, unusual for me, as I usually treasure those captive hours, having learned to soothe my moderate flying anxiety by losing myself in a book. Instead, I ordered a glass of white wine from the flight attendant and turned out my overhead light. During that entire three-hour trip back to Edmonton, my eyes remained fixed on the window, on the stars and the moon in the cloudless indigo sky. On infinity.

When we landed in Edmonton, I was one of the first people to disembark. Inside the terminal, the customs officer asked about the purpose of my trip and I responded with one word: pleasure. Within minutes, I was in a taxi. Except for our hungry and somewhat lonely cat, my house was empty because my husband was on a golf trip to California, and none of our three children have lived with us for almost a decade. As I stood in my silent kitchen, I pulled the pamphlet from Taliesin West out of my purse and knew I'd always remember that I'd been in Arizona when I became an orphan, when I lost my second parent twenty-five years after losing the first. That phrase still feels strange. Saying "I lost my mother" sounds as if I somehow misplaced her, forgot where I put her, did not know her where-abouts. As if I could find her again.

I was calm as I unpacked my suitcase and put my clothes in the laundry hamper, calm as I brushed my teeth, washed my face, and climbed into bed. Once under the covers, with the cat curled up against my back, I cried myself to sleep. My mother was dead, and as the eldest of her five orphaned children, I was next in line.

The next morning, approximately eighteen hours after my mother's death, I woke up to an empty refrigerator. I made some herbal tea and fed the cat. Knowing that my phone would start ringing soon as the family began the task of planning a funeral, I threw on my jacket and headed to the grocery store. While I was paying for my bread and yogurt at the checkout, the cashier asked if I wanted a bag for my items. What I meant to say was no. What came out was, "My mother died yesterday."

The words were out of my mouth before I could stop them, beyond my control. They were like water overflowing a sink. It was a relief to say them out loud, but it was odd to say them to a complete stranger, someone from outside my circle, someone with no knowledge of my family's dynamics. A weak laugh escaped me as I tried to take the words back.

"I apologize. I don't know why I said that."

The cashier smiled. "It's okay. My grandmother died last year. I know how you feel. And I'm sorry about your mother."

Grief is sometimes more easily shared with strangers than with intimates.

Perforated Hearts

I keep a file of unsent special occasion cards in my desk drawer
at home. The plain manila folder I store them in bulges with
unused greeting cards, such as the Father's Day card I should
have sent to my dad the year he died. I can't remember exactly
why I didn't mail it. My parents had recently separated after
a thirty-seven-year marriage, so it's possible that I was a little
angry with both of them. Or perhaps I simply didn't have
his new address. In all likelihood, the card lay on my kitchen
counter for several days until it was too late to put it in the mail.
As I placed it in my card file, I thought I'd be able to use it the
following year.

Some cards are in that file because I picked them out of
the store's display rack and they stayed in my hand. Rarely do
I walk away from my favourite greeting-card store with fewer
than three or four cards, most of which I don't need at the time.
I might like the drawing on the front, or how the colours evoke
the card's message. I might like the font used for the words,
but only if the words are few. If I pick out a card and find a long
verse in flowing script on the inside, I close it at once and put it

back on the shelf, unread. None of the cards in my file contain many words.

Several years ago, in an effort to declutter my office, I went on a rampage. I spent a whole afternoon clearing out any papers threatening to overtake my desk and file drawers. One of the files I went through was the one holding all my unused greeting cards. One of the cards I sent to the recycling bin was the Father's Day card I'd never sent. As soon as it was gone, I missed it. That was when I knew my card file had evolved from being merely a place to store extra cards into something else. It had become a private compilation of mainstream consumer culture that resonated with me in one way or another. I don't purge it any more.

One of the items in my collection ended up there many years ago after I'd sent my daughter out on a hurried shopping mission, back when she was a teenager with a brand-new driver's license. We were having an informal dinner party that evening, and late in the afternoon I realized that I needed a birthday card for one of our guests. Nothing in my file was appropriate, so I sent my daughter on a quick shopping trip. In what I see now as an endearing inherited trait, she came back from the store with two or three cards, including one that remains in my file to this day.

The front features three comic-strip style illustrations, each one showing an egg-headed cartoon figure wearing a suit and a bow tie. Drawing number one has the cartoon figure holding an egg. He looks at the viewer and says, "OK, one more time. This is your BRAIN." Drawing number two has the cartoon figure holding a frying pan in the air. The egg is now resting on a table. The cartoon figure says, "This is the effect of the AGEING PROCESS on your brain." Drawing number three shows that the cartoon figure has slammed the frying pan down onto the egg. Shell, albumen, and yolk detritus appear in all corners of the frame. The inside of the card has no illustration, only a caption that reads, "Any questions?"

I think I laughed for a full ten minutes the first time I read this card. My husband and my daughter laughed, too. But we also knew that we wouldn't be using it that night. Or at all. Sometimes my daughter and I still laugh when we talk about that card. But it's a different kind of laughter now, deeper, more solemn. In the decades since that day, we've had both Alzheimer's disease and dementia strike our family. I'm glad I have that card in my file, so that no one else could buy it and actually give it to someone. In vain, I hope it was the only one of its kind.

My favourite card in that manila file has also been in there for a long time. In fact, it might have been the reason I started the file in the first place. It's a Valentine's Day card I purchased back in the days before cellphones eliminated pay phones from street corners. I never had any intention of sending it to anyone. I bought it because once I'd read it, my hand would not put it back on the shelf. The cover illustration is a drawing of a dishevelled woman. She has yellow hair and a blue boa scarf around her neck that doesn't quite conceal her cartoon cleavage. She isn't young and she isn't old. Between her thumb and her forefinger she has a quarter that she is holding up to eye level. Looking straight out at the viewer, not smiling, not frowning, she says, "If I had a quarter for every romantic Valentine's Day I've had..." On the inside of the card, she finishes her sentence: "I could make a phone call."

Every time I dig around in my card file, I read this one and laugh. Occasionally I wonder why it speaks to me so much. I wasn't unhappy or lonely in my life when I bought it. In fact, I was contentedly content. I think it's the fullness, the world-weary ennui of the "I could make a phone call" line that made this card stay in my hand the day I found it. Even content-edly content, the middle-aged me was already indifferent to

February's celebration of love, was already wondering if there was ever a time in my life when I didn't think of Valentine's Day as a puerile occasion of little substance.

Yet I couldn't have always felt like that. Surely a younger version of me once yearned for the gush and rush of publicly declared romantic love. When I think back, I try to pinpoint the moment in my life when a younger me shifted her vision of love's annual day to an assessment similar to my yellow-haired, boa-bedecked cartoon friend. But I can't affix it to any event or time. My Valentine's Day apathy merely evolved.

I do welcome mid-February's love-fest as a temporary distraction from winter's unceasing hold. But, if it were up to me, I'd rename the occasion. Instead of Valentine's Day, I'd call it Big Red Heart Day in honour of the millions of those icons sold and exchanged in the middle of the year's shortest month. Or maybe Perforated Heart Day because so many of those rounded red shapes are punctured by arrows.

Valentine's Day falls on the fifty-fifth day of winter in the northern hemisphere. For Canadians, it's the first special occasion of the year since the beginning of January. A take-it-as-it-falls day, Valentine's Day doesn't move to the nearest Monday or Friday to create a long weekend. Whatever day of the week February the fourteenth hits is it. And it's a get-up-and-go-to-work day, especially if your place of employment happens to be in the restaurant industry, or at a florist shop, or behind the counter in a chocolaterie. Love sells, so people have to work.

When I stand in a greeting-card store in February, I get no sense of the history of Valentine's Day. No cards show images of St. Valentine, whoever he was. His history is murky. He may or may not have been one of the several saintly men named Valentine who may or may not have lived in Rome in the third century. And one of these men may or may not have been a priest who was executed on February fourteenth. Apparently his crime was that he cured his jailer's daughter of blindness, and then attempted to convert her father to Christianity. Myths passed down through the centuries tell us that on the night before his execution, the doomed priest sent an endearing note to his jailer's daughter, perhaps giving him the distinction of composing the very first Valentine's Day card. But none of this shows on the modern-day cards available almost everywhere as soon as all leftover Christmas merchandise disappears from store shelves. Love sells—mythic history not so much.

The history of Valentine's Day is not limited to ancient Rome. In the courtly love era of Geoffrey Chaucer's England, a barely post-medieval, plague-filled, war-ravaged period known as the late Middle Ages, February's love messages were hand-crafted missives, erotic exchanges shared in secret between married people and their lovers. A husband without a lover would go out and find one. A wife without a lover would simply have a night off; perhaps that was the best kind of Valentine's Day for her. Or perhaps she spent the night yearning for the sound of galloping hooves indicating that a love note speared on a lance was about to appear at her turret window.

The word "forever" is found on many Valentine's Day cards, as if love is a timeless, unchanging entity. And yes, falling in love has been part of human life since the beginning, but only in the last few centuries has marrying for love been a standard of Western life. Back in courtly England, marriage was not a romantic union. More often than not, it was a business arrange-ment, an enterprise intended to benefit a family's social and economic standing, a negotiation in which the female was the traded commodity. Indeed, back in Chaucer's time, love and marriage were considered incompatible. In one of the most famous love stories from that era, the lovely Heloise is said to have refused to marry her theologian lover Abelard even after the birth of their child, not only because marriage would damage his religious career, but because it would also diminish their love.

Why is a Valentine's Day heart rounded and red? Why is love symbolized by two ear-shaped halves linked together, one facing forwards and one flipped backwards? Some people say that the shape of the symbolic heart comes from the silhouette of two swans facing each other, touching their beaks together. Others claim that it comes from a vague replication of what an actual human heart looks like when removed from the body and plunked down on a cold metal table. Still others argue that it comes from the shape of female genitalia. Whatever its source, the Valentine's Day heart takes much abuse. It melts, burns, and breaks.

Our physical hearts cannot withstand such abuse. If they melt, burn, or break, we die. Usually, our symbolic hearts survive all the melting and the breaking. They may shatter and harden, but we will still breathe and our blood will still flow. If our physical hearts undergo the same trauma, we call an ambulance. This is not to say that the symbolic heart and the physical heart aren't connected. Emotions felt by our symbolic hearts can make our real hearts beat faster or slower, or even skip a beat, thanks to signals from our brains. Such is the complexity of the walking, talking, thinking, feeling corporeal instruments we live in.

I sympathize with my real heart and the incessant work it does without requiring instructions from me. We never have to tell our hearts what to do or how to go about it. They already know to slow down when we sleep and work harder when we climb a steep hill. They already know to pump red oxygenated blood out through the body, to receive in return blue oxygen-depleted blood, to disperse that tired blood to the lungs for oxygen replenishment, to receive it back newly reddened, and pump it out again. Our bodies are ever-flowing bloody rivers, our hearts both the source and the destination of that flow.

My heart works at a moderate rate when I roam up and down the aisles of almost any grocery or department store in early February. At that time of year, the shelves are flush with hearts. Red velvet hearts. Pink flowery hearts. Deep burgundy hearts trimmed with white lace. In a poem titled "Variations on the Word Love," written back in the early 1980s, Margaret Atwood says that we use the word to fill gaps. The poem situates love as a word now impoverished because we've given it too much trite work to do. We fling it around a lot. We love things—cars, food, wine, hotels, puppies, and clothing. As the poem progresses, Atwood changes her approach and observes that, as a word, love is too small for its real work, its meagre collection of letters far too inadequate to express the power of a feeling that can have us floating several feet off the ground one minute and flatten us like road-kill the next. We utter this short four-letter word both carefully and carelessly. Maybe we should restrict its use. Maybe we should ban its application to inanimate objects. Maybe we should use it only when referring to someone or something that also has a heart.

A few years ago, just after the Christmas season, when department and grocery store aisles first began to bulge with fancy chocolate assortments and fluffy heart-shaped candy boxes, I stood looking at it all for many minutes. I wondered how people could be so easily manipulated into spending their money on superficial love tokens. But that question faded even as I stood there. Perhaps because I watched numerous shoppers walk up to that garish inventory and spend a long time selecting the perfect lacy, frilly, velvety valentine for their chosen one, lingering as they picked up, examined, and rejected one after the other. Perhaps the small smile I saw on an older man's face as he tucked his selected token under his arm and shuffled off to the checkout convinced me that Big Red Heart Day might serve more than our economy.

"Love Me Tender" sings Elvis in his eternal after-death life. But romantic love doesn't stay tender. It gets rough and choppy, lost and found, old and then young again. Twice I made that impossible wedding day promise to feel forever exactly the same way about my beloved as I did in that heady moment. Both times I meant it. I failed to keep that promise the first time. The second time around, I managed to learn that feelings can change in ways that don't sink a relationship, that a few turbulent skids on the marriage road don't necessarily mean an appointment with a divorce lawyer.

As a kid, the most memorable part of my childhood Valentine's Days was the night before, when I'd sit at our kitchen table with a pair of blunt-ended scissors in my right hand, even though I'm left-handed. Left-handed scissors were hard to come by back then, and no doubt a luxury our family couldn't afford, even though three out of the seven people living in our house were left-handed. We owed our odd-handedness to my paternal grandfather, a man of Scottish heritage who wore a suit and tie every single day until he was almost ninety-five, and the staff at his nursing home managed to convince him that he was fully dressed even without a tie. When my grandfather started school back in the early twentieth century, he was forced to learn penmanship with his awkward right hand. The same thing happened to my father a generation later. These events condemned both men to lifetimes of illegible handwriting.

I don't think it mattered to my right-handed mother which hand I used for any task, as long as I was doing something useful. However, when his left-handed eldest child started school, my father participated in his first, and perhaps last, parent-teacher meeting on my behalf. Although I know that rigid social thinking about the supremacy of right-handedness had already begun to ease, I like to think it was because of Dad's intervention that I was allowed to write with my left hand. Nevertheless, the world I lived in was, and in many ways still is, predominantly right-handed, and even though I was permitted to write with it, I still had to abandon my left hand for many things, including scissoring.

My right-handed mother and my left-handed father may have given each other Valentine's Day cards, but I don't remember what those parental tokens of affection looked like. If they did, my mother would have displayed the cards for a few days, first on the buffet in the dining room, and then upstairs on the dresser in their bedroom. Finally, they'd be stored for a few months or years, in a drawer someplace in the house, but not in the kitchen. The kitchen was for preparation—of food and Valentines.

I do remember the Valentines I gave to my school friends. They were the same ones I received in return. In fact, if I had to go shopping for schoolyard Valentine's Day cards right now, I could probably find the identical ones we used decades ago. Valentines haven't changed much over the years of my life. On the weekend before February fourteenth, while out doing her Saturday grocery shopping, my mother always bought one of those oversized rectangular booklets of cut-out Valentines. Sometimes she'd splurge and buy a more expensive booklet made out of stiffer cardboard. These had perforated edges around each card so scissors weren't required. I could just punch them out and print my friends' names on them. But sometimes the perforations were tough and didn't separate well. Sometimes they tore into the pretty fronts of the cards. And sometimes they left little tufts along the edges that I thought spoiled their look. I never told Mom that I liked the cheaper ones better, that I enjoyed the feel of curving my right-handed scissors around those red shapes. My scissored hearts had smooth clean perfect edges. The perforated hearts were ragged and marred.

I no longer fall into the middle-aged category, my life having progressed past the point where I can continue to convince myself that I'm only halfway through it. These days, as the fourteenth of February draws nearer, I find myself bemused by all the fuss. But I still ponder the purpose of Valentine's Day. Not the obvious economic purpose that serves our commodity world so well, but the reason our communal psyche needs it. A mental image has taken root in my mind, one in which our hearts are fragile eggs living in chaotic places where menacing frying pans lurk around every corner. Maybe Valentine's Day is the reassuring demonstration our insecure culture needs, the collective hug we require, a reminder that simple love does exist in a complicated world.

Nowadays, my husband and I don't put much emphasis on Valentine's Day. If we get each other a card, that's fine. If we forget, that's okay, too. In our first years together, I always wanted to go out for dinner on the fourteenth of February. And my husband obliged me. But gradually we began to resent that our favourite restaurants had different menus and higher prices on that one night. These days both of us would much rather stay home, share a bottle of wine, and cook a meal together. He looks after the protein while I build a salad. Sometimes we even put on a little music, maybe something with a good, swingy beat that gets us dancing around our kitchen. When we do that, somewhere in a corner of my mind, I see my left-handed father dancing with my right-handed mother, their scarred marred hearts only inches apart as they move around a kitchen that no longer exists, swaying to a song no one sings anymore.

Giant Bunnies
Don't Deliver Chocolate Eggs

The house I grew up in contained a diverse collection of footwear, in seven different sizes, for all seasons and occasions. During the winter, when the piles at the back door grew large and hazardous, my mother would toss them down the basement stairs one by one. Then she'd follow them down and make a line at the bottom, a long row of pairs from biggest to smallest, tallest to shortest. Inevitably, she'd end up with at least one shoe or boot that didn't have a mate. These orphans went into a corner to wait until their wayward partners eventually turned up.

During the long Winnipeg winters, we went outside whenever we could. We went ice-skating and took rides across the football field behind our house on our fancy new snowmobile. I don't know how we got that machine. It just showed up one day. My father might have won it in a sales contest at his office. Everyone said Dad was a natural salesman, that he could sell snowballs to Eskimos or suspenders to Mennonites. It's hard to believe now that people actually said things like that during everyday kitchen table chitchat, but they did. Anyway, it would have been most unusual for either of my parents to buy anything as extravagant as that. My father had to have gotten it for free somehow.

Other than those two activities, I remember spending much of winter indoors, looking out through frosted window panes with their crazy crystal shapes blocking our views of the ice fog outside. We'd chuckle when visitors, unaccustomed to the polar air, gasped the first time they felt it hit their lungs. Frigid air burns on its way into the body.

Each winter the day would finally come, usually sometime in March, when I'd shuffle home from school with my winter boots unfastened, my coat unbuttoned, my scarf untied, my woolly hat thrown into my book bag, and my mitts dangling from the strings threaded through my sleeves. As warmth gradually returned to the prairie sun, Winnipeg's high snowbanks receded and puddles of all sizes materialized on the streets and sidewalks. Soon, my winter boots could join the lineup at the bottom of the stairs, and I'd head off to school in my galoshes. My walks home would then take even longer because no puddle could go by undisturbed.

I can't imagine my paternal grandmother ever stomping through a puddle unless it was completely unavoidable. Even in the daytime, she was always dressed as if she were off to have lunch at Winnipeg's stately Fort Garry Hotel; her sturdy but stylish shoes were definitely not puddle-jumpers. Her family was Irish, but not the born-in-Ireland Irish. Granny was born in Lethbridge, Alberta. Her father, my great-grandfather, wasn't born in Ireland either, but somewhere in Ontario. Nevertheless, their family name was one of those "O'" words, and my grandmother insisted on her Irishness. This meant that sometime in the first two weeks of March, my mother, Granny's dutiful daughter-in-law, would buy a St. Patrick's Day card, inscribe it, address the envelope, and lick an eight- or ten-cent stamp for the corner. Often I was the one who walked down the street to the mailbox to start that card on its journey into my grand-mother's hands. I was always warned not to drop the envelope in a puddle.

I recently read that St. Patrick's Day is the friendliest holiday of the year. I think that has a lot to do with green. Green beer, green faces, and green rivers. Green, the friendly cool colour, the colour of spring. St. Patrick's Day is a minor seasonal marker, a fun occasion in which people of all origins go to the pub and misbehave with impunity. It's more a party than any-thing else, a short rest stop on the way to something bigger and better, spring's defining holiday celebration: Easter.

In our house, Easter was not nearly as exciting as Christmas, what with all that heady shopping frenzy, the letters to Santa Claus, and the secret caches of presents hidden under beds or behind locked closet doors. But Easter was still a day we awaited with eager anticipation. From January to March, the wearers of all those shoes and boots endured—with as much patience as we could muster—the three-month gap between candy canes and chocolate eggs, between stockings placed on the floor in front of our tinsel-filled tree (we didn't have a mantel to hang them from) and the lineup of purple and yellow straw baskets on the mahogany dining-room table.

As a kid, I believed the Santa Claus story because at least he was human. I willingly suspended my disbelief about his flying sleigh, those soaring reindeer, and the fact that even a five-year-old could see that it was impossible for anyone to deliver presents to every house in the world, land on all those rooftops, and slide down all those chimneys. Besides, our house didn't have a fireplace, and I knew that the chimney on our roof led directly to the furnace. When I mentioned this to my parents, they said that Santa jumped off our roof and came in the front door. They also told me not to ask that question in front of my younger siblings.

My belief in Santa Claus lasted as long as I wanted it to. One year, when I was seven or eight, I informed my parents, as they were enjoying their evening cocktail at the kitchen table, that Santa couldn't possibly be real, that I knew they bought all our presents at the Hudson's Bay store downtown. They said I was growing up, and admitted I was right. My mother also corrected my claim about her shopping habits: not everything came from the Bay. She also ordered from the Eaton's catalogue. That night after I went to bed, I remember being a little miffed that my parents had lied to me all the years of my life. And then I felt a little guilty about being miffed at my parents for wanting me to believe in Santa Claus. Being a kid is difficult at times. We have to let our parents have their moments of parenting fun.

I've never been to Easter Island, but I've seen pictures of those bizarre, morose stone statues that stand on its shore. According to Wikipedia, Easter Island was "encountered" on Easter Sunday in 1792. A Dutch explorer found it even though it is located in an isolated part of the Pacific Ocean somewhere between New Zealand and Argentina. That's a little like trying to find your last quarter, the one that slipped out of your frozen fingers and disappeared into a four-foot high snow drift just as you were plugging it into a parking meter.

Today Easter Island is known not only for those giant stone faces, but also as an environment that once had trees. Those trees not only had birds living in their branches, they also provided the raw material for building ships to sail away on, or at least rafts to help with fishing. Lessons learned from Easter Island's history are that no tall trees = no birds = no shipbuilding = a bad conservationist reputation.

I've often thought that my mother was the original conservationist. She was recycling before the word "environment" came to define our relationship with the outside world. Even in the fifties, she was saving paper bags and washing out jam jars. She cut up the Christmas cards we received the year before and used them as gift tags on our presents. Back then, this wasn't known as recycling. It was called being thrifty.

Our family looked forward to Easter as the moment of release back into a more welcoming outside world. Despite T. S. Eliot's famous claim that "April is the cruellest month," I'm of the mind that March is meaner. Its very name suggests movement. But its march towards the first day of spring often comes to a complete halt. The biggest blizzard I've ever been in hit Winnipeg in March 1966, and ever since then, I've distrusted March days. They can turn nasty in an instant.

For me, spring doesn't arrive until Easter. That's when I'm willing to believe that winter has succumbed at last, that the annual softening season has begun, that my daily routine is about to shift from long dark evenings to after-dinner wakefulness, from hibernation to emergence. But Easter, like Hemingway's Paris, is a moveable entity that requires an annual adjustment.

Among its holiday cousins, Easter is unique for two reasons. First, it's a reverse long weekend, because the day off falls on a Friday rather than a Monday. Second, it's a mobile holiday, the one major celebration of the year that doesn't have a fixed day, the one holiday that provokes the annual question, "When is Easter this year anyway?"

The method for determining Easter's spot on the calendar is so complicated that it rivals the one for converting Fahrenheit into Celsius. (I've tried to memorize that formula for years, giving up only when I discovered an app on my cellphone that does it for me.) Establishing a date for Easter is much more difficult. On one level, it has a loose rotation of early one year and late the next. On another level entirely beyond my comprehension, the calculation involves the phases of the moon, the cycle of the spring equinox and the summer solstice, as well as the number of Sundays that fall between March twenty-second and April twenty-fifth. I should hire the person who came up with that formula to balance my monthly budget.

In the two cities I've called home in my life, Winnipeg and Edmonton, Easter and spring are no guarantees of warmth. April blizzards often leave our budding tulips poking through wet heavy snow. On the flood plains, prairie residents watch warily as rivers rise up their banks, bloated with runoff and rain. Yet we take whatever these months bring because when it finally arrives, spring is, in the words of e e cummings, "mud-luscious" and "puddle-wonderful."

And it's one of the most common themes in the literary world. Sometimes spring appears in a story as a subtle reference, such as when an adept writer like Margaret Atwood interrupts a tense narrative moment by having an adult daughter ask her ageing mother if the crocuses are up yet. This conversation takes place in a story called "Significant Moments in the Life of My Mother," which opens Atwood's short story collection, *Bluebeard's Egg*. The egg in that title has nothing to do with Easter.

At other times, the writerly use of spring is anything but subtle, acting as both the topic of the work and its subtext. The "mud-luscious" cummings poem "in Just/ spring" depicts game-playing, puddle-jumping children frolicking on the brink of their adolescent years, unaware that they are about to move from the spring of their lives into the complications of their summer seasons.

In more prosaic work, spring reading brings items from sports writers using words like exhibition, training camp, and curveball. Economic analysts watch for rising markets. Speechwriters working for politicians prefer composing material for spring elections, not only because of better voter turnout, but also because of general seasonal optimism. No matter what's going on in the world, spring suggests an upward trend. And it hosts Easter.

Besides the Easter Bunny and Santa Claus, the other fantasy figure parents introduce to their children is the Tooth Fairy. I don't know what season it was when I lost my first tooth. I think it might have been spring because I was at the grocery store with my mother, and I sense that I was feeling light, like I was outside without a winter jacket for the first time in a long while.

From the outset, I was suspicious of the Tooth Fairy because I could not picture a little Tinkerbell flying around with a sack of coins on her back. Surely the sack would interfere with her wings? At the checkout counter, after paying for our groceries, Mom asked for some nickels in her change. "Someone just lost a tooth," she said to the cashier, who nodded knowingly. The next morning, I didn't take me long to figure out where the nickel I found under my pillow had come from. But it was a nickel, so who was I to question who put it there?

The Easter Bunny began as a seventeenth-century hare that somehow morphed into the cuddly rabbit we know today. Some have speculated that the fertile hare became an Easter symbol because it's a hermaphrodite, but that doesn't make sense to me. Earthworms are hermaphrodites too, and we don't have an Easter Earthworm.

In Sweden, they have an Easter Tree, which is not a tree, but a handful of willow twigs decorated with colourful feathers and displayed in vases. That sounds much more labour-efficient than erecting an entire tree, plastic or otherwise, and spending several hours hanging sparkly lights, balls, and tinsel on it. I know I've just conflated my holidays, but you get my point; and I think I would like Sweden. Apparently, the Swedes also have an Easter Hag, an old woman who wears a headscarf and an apron and drinks an inordinate amount of coffee. I think the Easter Hag is the most believable imaginary figure I've ever heard of.

At home in Winnipeg, we had the Easter Bonnet. Back in the days when my mother took her family to church, I knew that the Easter Bonnet referred to the whole darn outfit, not just the hat. And I knew that each year, my mother would try to spruce up her family for our appearance in the Easter Parade, which wasn't really a parade, but a procession up the church sidewalk or aisle, taken at a strolling pace so that everyone had plenty of time to see all aspects of the Easter Bonnet. Unless the weather brought rain or snow, in which case we stayed home.

Our household was Anglican. I grew up with a mother who went to church on a regular basis, and a father who didn't go to church at all. When my siblings and I were young, my mother took us with her each week. As the years went by, herding all her children out of the house every Sunday morning became increasingly difficult. Sometimes it just wasn't worth the effort. Sometimes we all got to stay home and have a big eggy breakfast together. As the years passed, the big eggy breakfast won out completely.

Before we got to Easter Sunday, however, we had to go through Lent, the period of forty days leading up to Easter. This is a time of denial, traditionally a fast of some kind. I have read that the orthodox practice of Lent forbids eggs in the house and demands abstinence from meat and dairy. We were not exactly strict observers of these details. Our refrigerator was rarely without eggs and bacon. Still, on Sundays leading up to Lent, our minister would stress that it was an important period, a time for self-evaluation, self-improvement, and, of course, repentance.

When I went to church, I sat beside my mother and wondered about all this repentance I was supposed to be doing. I thought I was a relatively good kid; in fact, I couldn't think of a single thing I'd done wrong. Surely sticking my tongue out at my little brother couldn't possibly require anything as serious as repentance.

My mother took the minister's words to heart, and attempted to enforce Lent in her resistant household, with her own variations. For Mom, the Lenten denial wasn't necessarily restricted to food. She told me that for those forty days, I should give up something that was important to me. One year I said I would give up chewing on the eraser at the end of my pencil. My mother was not impressed. The next year, I went back to food, and gave up eating our usual Wednesday night dinner of liver and onions. This did not go over well either. Mom didn't believe that giving up liver was a noble sacrifice on my part.

Although she tried to instill religion in her children, Mom was very practical about her parenting priorities. She was firm about some rules. We were not to physically maim each other. Pulling each other's hair, or biting a sibling were punishable offenses. But a busy parent has only so much time for discipline, and in order to keep us physically safe, my mother let her Lenten efforts lapse, although she always did admonish me for chewing on the end of my pencil.

I'm a lapsed church-goer. Only recently did I discover that Easter also has something called Eastertide, a fifty-day period following the Easter celebration during which each Sunday is a symbolic feast day. I have no memory of any Eastertide in our house. As far as I was concerned, after I'd eaten all the chocolate eggs the giant bunny had left in my straw basket, after we'd eaten our Easter Sunday dinner of baked ham and scalloped potatoes, it was all over. I usually had Easter Monday off school, but Dad always went back to work that day because it wasn't a holiday for him.

Which brings me, finally you might say, back to that rabbit. Even as a little girl, I was skeptical about the Easter Bunny. I never did believe the story. A giant rabbit with a giant toothy smile carrying a giant basket with an endless supply of foiled-covered chocolate eggs? I might have been a kid, but I wasn't stupid. Besides, I knew that the purple and yellow straw baskets that held our candy eggs on Easter Sunday morning spent the rest of the year on the top shelf of my mother's bedroom closet.

Yet I grew up and did the same thing with my own children. I told them the same stories, went through the same rituals that perpetuate the Easter Bunny, Santa Claus, and Tooth Fairy myths. But I didn't try very hard. At the first sign of skepticism from them, I was happy to let the fantasies fall apart. As a parent, I found it hard to lie to my kids, to put much stock in these imaginary, gift-bearing, impossible-to-believe characters. I was relieved to let each ruse go. Then, as my children reached the age of young adulthood, and the big holidays became easier without the mandatory myth management, I was surprised to find that I missed jolly old Santa and the Easter Bunny—just a little. I told myself this was nonsense, and berated myself for whimsical softness towards manufactured magic.

Still, for several years I took a hard line, dismissing these likable lies as doing more harm than good by teaching children to distrust what their parents tell them. Now I'm softening a little, realizing that our mythical characters are as much for the parents as the kids, that we keep them alive in part because of our nostalgic yearning to return to where we came from. Nostalgia lives in the impossible notion that we can start again, maybe have an opportunity to fix a few of the mistakes we made along the way—regain time wasted, take back words hastily spoken, and share thoughts we kept to ourselves until it was too late. I suppose that makes nostalgia a little like repentance.

Gym Interrupted, Again

As spring approaches, I usually purge. Along with the longer days comes a need to declutter. Unused, neglected objects weigh heavy on me. My psyche feels tethered by too many boxes of items I rarely use, so I start going through closets and cupboards. I create piles. I drive to the Eco Station and the Goodwill drop-off site. With each trip, I feel lighter.

One spring, I found myself sitting on my bedroom floor, surrounded by heaps of old workout clothing I'd acquired over the last few decades: impossibly small shorts, striped tights, teeny tank tops, and even leg warmers, all of which had adorned my body in a gymnasium setting at one time or other. One by one, I held the items up in front of me and looked in the mirror. I tried to visualize each one on my body. Then I tried to visualize the body that fit into them. I was surprised by how small I once was. And even more surprised to remember that I'd always thought of myself as a little too big. But I wasn't surprised at how prevailing social attitudes about the female body sink into even the most resistant of minds, even mine.

My eclectic clothing collection suggested that I'd been a longtime, even dedicated, workout devotee. This is not entirely accurate. My workout regimen has always been subject to interruptions. I lapse often. After any prolonged absence, I'm inevitably daunted by the prospect of stepping through the door of a gym again. I know that inside I'll find well-toned gym people operating the complicated equipment with ease, making their workouts look effortless. Once I manage to propel myself into a gym, I tiptoe past everyone, eyes down, hoping I look as invisible as I feel.

Whenever I return after a prolonged exercise hiatus, I start out with a group class because I know I need someone to tell me what to do. Arriving at a gym without a plan is like going on a road trip without a map. I position myself at the back, trying not to see the small smiles between veterans who've watched each other over a period of time, and are confident about their status in the fitness hierarchy. As the class progresses, I work to keep my facial expression impassive, whether or not I make it to the end of each exercise set. I do my best to ignore the pleading voice in my head: *Please don't make me do anything conspicuous. What's with all these mirrors? We're going to do what? She's got to be kidding.* Once that inner voice grows too loud to be silenced, I know that my sporadic exercise regimen is in danger of lapsing once again.

My first set of workout clothes was the junior high school uniform I had to wear to Phys Ed class: a crisp white cotton shirt—with a collar and buttons, no less—and navy-blue shorts with built-in bloomers designed to guard against any glimpses of underwear. My mother loathed that uniform even more than I did. It was one more thing she had to buy on a constrained budget. I also remember her saying that those ridiculous shorts bled blue into the rest of her laundry.

Our gym teacher insisted on a neat appearance, so I often had to retuck that stupid blouse into my shorts as I hauled myself around the gender-partitioned gym. We did our push-ups, jumping jacks, and other uncomfortable calisthenics while listening to the noises from the other side of the flimsy wall, where the boys played their games. The great guffaws of laughter we heard from their side produced insatiable curiosity on ours. They sounded like they were having much more fun than we were. They sounded like they didn't know or care that we could hear them.

Other than Phys Ed class, I didn't do much exercise in high school: I played a little badminton and made the cheerleading squad for the community football team. After high school, I don't remember participating in any formal exercise at all. Those were the days when exercise happened in the regular course of daily life, the days before computers.

About five years after I graduated from high school, I went to a yoga class with a new friend. This session was very unlike the yoga classes of today: practiced in beautiful rooms with soothing music playing in the background, incense tantalizing the nostrils, and glowing tealights gently illuminating a warm hardwood floor. Today, we wear specially designed pants made of fabric that helps us with our downward dogs, and matching tops that sit easily on our bodies, move with us into our tree and warrior poses.

For that long-ago first yoga experience, my friend and I went to a large gym complex on a military base on a dark January night. I wore baggy shorts and a sloppy T-shirt. We changed our clothes in a cold locker room with a cement floor. As our instructor led us into the first poses, the only "music" we heard came from the beat of a basketball game going on next door. The only scents were of disinfectant and smelly old socks forgotten somewhere under the bleachers. The harsh glare from the mercury vapour lights up in the rafters did not gently illuminate anything.

After class, we changed back into our winter wear in the cold locker room. My friend glanced around at our yoga classmates, now in various states of undress. She whispered in my ear: *There really are no perfect bodies, are there?*

My relationship with gym yoga was interrupted by motherhood. It's funny about motherhood: during pregnancy, everything was about my body. Afterwards, the baby distracted all attention away from me. I only thought about my body when it interfered with what I had to do each day. Which was a lot. Having three children in two years (the second one turned out to be twins) meant that I didn't have much time, or need, to think about fitness.

During those years when my children were small, I occasionally spent an evening playing racquetball with a friend. Also a mother of twins, she was better at the game than me, but that didn't matter. All I wanted to do was beat the hell out of that ball for an hour or so, and then retreat to the nearest bar for a glass of wine. It was a night out. I didn't care what I looked like or what I wore; in fact, I considered myself lucky to reach into a laundry basket and find something that was both mine and clean. Style was the last thing on my mind.

Eventually, I joined a small neighbourhood gym, and worked a few aerobics classes into a schedule that by then included a full-time job and three children in elementary school. Those were the days of skinny striped headbands, funky leg warmers, and matching body suits; of that plague suffered by many aerobics fanatics—shin splints; of Gloria Gaynor's "I Will Survive" pounding out the beat. My favourite aerobics outfit was a bright royal-blue leotard I wore with pink leg warmers. I felt happy in it. Our cheery instructor choreographed our workouts into dance routines, and shouted out that we could do it, we could make it, we could shake it.

Our aerobics group came together for the exercise, but the shared coffee-times afterwards became equally important. Occasionally we gathered for social evenings, bringing with us our spouses, zesty appetizers, and common concerns about careers and children. Having had a few upheavals in my life—a divorce and a new marriage—this group became a welcome oasis for me, less about fitness and more about companionship, if only for a few hours a week.

Gradually, the aerobics phase of my life waned. Many of the people in our group, including me, drifted on to other things. Pressures on my time became increasingly difficult to manage, and gym activities fell out of my daily, and then my weekly, routine. Inevitably, I stopped going altogether.

I dealt with this interruption in my gym life by establishing a regular running routine. Three times a week, I headed down into my city's beautiful river valley, guiltily leaving my dog at home because the park by the river was off-limits to dogs, and my running feet always took me towards the river. My children could walk the dog. I had to run.

Despite living in a body that clearly wasn't built for running (short legs, low centre of gravity, bottom-heavy), I surprised myself with a physical endurance I didn't know I had. I also discovered that I am one of the slowest runners ever to lace up a far-too-expensive pair of training shoes. Starting out was painful, but once I got going, I was a human version of the Energizer Bunny stuck on low speed. I felt as if I could go forever.

Alas, my running career didn't last, but not because I didn't enjoy running. I did: I often felt the solitude was the best part of it, but the solitude also got in my way. Nobody expected me to show up. Nobody urged me to carry on. In the end, nobody but me noticed when I stopped doing it. I did, however, end up with fresh additions to my wardrobe: black running tights, a red windbreaker, various baseball caps, and several pairs of high-performance running shoes, one that even had an air pump in each heel.

As my motivation to run waned, I didn't ask myself why. Had I taken the time then to examine my exercise history, I might have noticed a pattern of starting and stopping, of engaging and withdrawing, of bravado and hesitation. But I didn't take stock of myself back then, and soon stopped making any attempts at physical fitness whatsoever. I chose wilful blindness, simply ignoring my body and avoiding gyms (and mirrors) entirely for a few years. I worked, socialized, raised my teenagers, and convinced myself that walking the dog would take care of any exercise I needed. Unsurprisingly, my fitness level deteriorated at a rate directly proportional to the larger clothing sizes I required.

A few years later, my husband bought me a treadmill for Christmas. It was well-used for a while, sometimes by me, more often by my daughters. But treadmills, like human bodies, need maintenance, and ours seemed to be a high-maintenance model. During prolonged periods of disrepair, it stood idle. I closed the door to the room it was in so I didn't see it every time I walked by.

More years passed. When our three young adults all moved out of the house, my husband and I decluttered our lives by having a huge garage sale. I sold the treadmill, and finally admitted that it was time to join a gym again. I found a new urban version downtown. There I discovered that things had changed in my absence. Gyms were now "fitness centres." A revolution had taken place while I wasn't paying attention. The biggest change was in the equipment. Cardio machines with stairs

and arm levers, racks of dumbbells and free weights, colourful
stability balls, and a plethora of odd-looking devices with pulley
systems filled every corner. Strange equipment and a multitude
of weight machines weren't the only new additions to the gym
world. Personal trainers had arrived. Brimming with confidence,
they led their charges through structured routines, feeding
them into the equipment like dough into pasta-machines:
plump and shapeless on entry, hopefully lean and flat coming
out the other end.

The cardio equipment was the most popular. Some gym-
goers seemed to spend hours on a treadmill, only to get off and
step immediately onto a cross-trainer or a stair-climber for yet
another hour. Water bottles and personal music devices had
become required accessories.

Televisions hung from the ceilings, placed at convenient
angles, so that visual distraction from exercise was everywhere:
news, soap operas, weather, sports, talk shows, and music
videos. All the noise of the outside world had entered the gym.

After a few months of regular attendance, I decided to
challenge myself, and booked some sessions with a friendly
personal trainer. She assessed my body and calculated my fat
mass—a disturbing experience for the self-deluded. After leading me through a few test exercises, she set up a program and
a schedule for us: once a week, I worked out with her; twice a
week, I followed our program on my own. To my surprise, I took
to this new regimen. I liked the balance, the expectation that
every seven days I worked with someone who told me how well
I was doing, who relied on me to have come to the gym at least
twice since our last meeting. Our program progressed like this
for several months.

During this time, I was largely oblivious to what went on
around me while I was working out. I didn't pay any attention to
who else was there, who was wearing what, or even what I was

wearing. I wore the most nondescript clothing possible: I didn't want to be distracted by fashion. Single-minded focus was my new mandate. As it turned out, I was oblivious even to the obvious. Eventually, my personal trainer had to draw my attention to her emerging condition: she was pregnant and would soon be taking an extended maternity leave.

Outwardly, I gave the expected response—a hug, motherly anecdotes about the joys to come. Inwardly, I was churlish: *What about me? How could you do this to me?* In retrospect, I hope my reaction was a little less self-absorbed than that. Beneath my dismay, I truly was happy for her. Ever gracious, she said that my routine needn't be disrupted, and offered to refer me to another trainer until she came back. I declined. I said I would be fine on my own.

A few months later, my personal trainer had a healthy baby boy, and all the gym people, me included, helped celebrate his arrival. After the excitement of the birth died down, I went to the gym exactly twice. Six months later, I cancelled my membership. Gym interrupted, again.

What followed was a particularly long period of physical stupor during which I resigned myself to inevitable decay. My workout clothes began to taunt me from the drawers they filled. I ignored them. I'm older now, I thought. I don't need to care as much about what I look like. This is what happens to everyone. Why fight it?

One day, I found myself in a clothing store fitting room trying on blue jeans. I've always worn blue jeans. They're my go-to comfort clothing. But I no longer had any that fit me. I'm not saying I was huge, just bigger than I'd ever been when I wasn't pregnant. Three of the fitting-room walls had mirrors on them, so I had a three-way view of myself in the six pairs of jeans I tried on, two different styles, three sizes each. None of them fit me. Not one pair. They were all too tight around my thighs. And if they were big enough to accommodate my butt, the waist was huge. I left still attired in the stretchy sweatpants I'd worn into the store.

So I found another new gym. Everyone in it was young. Everyone was beautiful and smiling. Almost everyone in it was slim. That may or may not have been the case, but that's what I saw when I walked in. Luckily, on that first day, I ran into an old friend. We squealed and hugged. Most of the time, I have great disdain for adult women who squeal like adolescent girls in public, but every once in a while I'm one of them.

My friend told me that she'd started exercising again because she refused to succumb to the old woman who was threatening to take over her body. I recognized that old woman immediately. She was inside me, too. My friend and I established a regular gym routine together. A mutual friend joined us, so sometimes we were three. Once more, people expected me to walk through a gym door—or rather a "health club" door, fitness centres-cum-gyms having been renamed yet again in my absence.

My now more-than-middle-aged body responded positively. I liked my reunion with the machines, the regular routine, the chats with my friends as we walked on the treadmills, the challenges we threw out to each other, the times we fell off the stability balls doubled over with laughter, disrupting the normally stoic health-club atmosphere. I was back. I was a gym person once more. Soon I booked a few sessions with a new personal trainer to add more depth to my workout routine. She and I hit it off immediately. Living life in my body was good again.

Eventually, I started to look around my health club. Things were different, somehow. For a while I couldn't figure out what it was. Then it hit me. It wasn't the physical space that had changed this time. It was the people. Gym people now came in all shapes and ages. Old and young, big and small, male and female circulated in, on, and around the equipment, taking turns, sometimes nodding and friendly, sometimes cool and remote.

On many of these varied bodies, one physical feature had gained unmistakable prominence: cleavage. Set off by fashionable new gym attire, the female breast was busting out all over the place. I found myself fascinated as shapely young women prepared for their workouts in the locker room, carefully settling their breasts into V-necked tops with built-in bras. They spent considerable time in front of the mirror before making their entrances into the public arena. It was as if they were prepping for a date rather than a workout.

Then my friend moved away. After she left, I kept going to the gym for a while, but then I let my training sessions expire, and eventually my gym visits came to a complete halt once again. Months passed with me ignoring the clean folded workout clothes sitting on top of my dresser. Then my phone rang one evening. It was my most recent personal trainer: *Where are you? Come back.* I couldn't think of a good reason not to, and she was so very nice to have called, so I did.

My experiences in these various exercise situations sometimes remind me of my old friend from that long-ago yoga class. Today she might have to admit that there are indeed some "perfect" bodies walking around. I see male physiques that are breathtaking in bulk, astonishing with their six-pack abs and rippled muscles. Yet, much as I appreciate attractive male bodies, it's often the females that draw my attention. When I see young women with incredibly slim hips and impossibly large breasts, I am first puzzled that this version of so-called physical perfection exists at all, and then perplexed at why women participate so avidly in its perpetuation.

To my voyeuristic eye, the most intriguing bodies are those that have "un-perfect" shapes, bodies that tell eloquent stories, lived-in bodies that don't deny their accumulated experiences, bodies that proudly wear their triumphs and their failures.

Whether I'm in a gym or outside in the world, as my body works up a sweat, my brain uses the time to mull. Workout time, it turns out, is good thinking time. For those of us fortunate enough to spend our lives in able bodies that we can take to the gym or the hiking trail, and for those of us fortunate enough that we don't have to spend every minute of our day ensuring our basic survival, life is full of choices. Life is also full of interruptions. People we care about move in and out of our days. We take jobs and we leave them. We start new endeavours and abandon old ones. We have children. They grow up and leave us. But the one relationship we have that isn't interrupted, at least until the day it ends forever, is the one we have with our bodies. They are the houses we live in.

In recent years, I've started to spend time swimming laps in a pool, a large public facility with swimming lanes, a play area, and a spa at one end. First I swim, then I warm my muscles in the hot tub. Always, I watch the people around me. The pool population seems slightly older than at the gym. Those who swim do so with languid strokes, reminiscent of stronger days.

Older bodies appreciate the helpful buoyancy of water. Older bodies do water aerobics. They bounce in chest-high water and walk or jog on the spot. They walk-jog in the swimming lanes. Sometimes, when the sun is hot, they wear floppy hats and sunglasses as they plow back and forth through the water. Some read books as they go. I was fascinated the first time I saw a woman walk-jog in a swim lane with a book in her hand. She saw me watching her, and laughed: "I have to do laps for half an hour, but I get bored."

Others skip the big pool altogether and head straight for the jets in the hot tub. Railings become very important at this stage of life. Late one afternoon, as the sun's daily retreat turned the western sky orange, I watched an elderly gentleman haul himself out of the spa, both hands on the railings. Each step up took several seconds, with a long pause in between. At the top, still hanging onto the railing, he aimed his feet at his waiting flip-flops. But he couldn't get them on. One errant flip-flop kept sliding away. Finally, he managed to pin it against the railing post and got a toehold on the sole. The second one went on a little easier. His feet shod, he reached for the towel hanging on his walker. Dried off, he draped the towel over his shoulders and started on his way. I watched as he left the pool, as he executed each step. First, he launched the walker forward. Then he moved his right foot up and dragged the left one beside it. At one point, his towel fell off his shoulders to the ground. I was nervous as he started to bend down to retrieve it, but a little girl standing nearby picked it up for him. She looked to be about six years old.

I watched that man all the way to the parking lot where his ride waited. I watched as he refused help from the driver, a middle-aged woman, perhaps his daughter. I watched as he stashed his walker in the back seat, and then folded himself into the front passenger seat. From hot tub to car, the whole exercise took twenty-five minutes. It was a workout.

After observing my once-strong mother fade into a sedentary inertia, I now have only one exercise rule. Keep moving. Movement is life. Sometimes I do my moving outside. Sometimes I do it in a gym. Sometimes I'm on my own. But I always make sure that I have a few dates where a buddy, an instructor, or a group is expecting me to show up. A mixture of solitude and companionship works best. I don't know why it took me so long to figure that out.

The Parent Days

I didn't want to write about Mother's Day. As I looked for my mother in the annual occasions we'd spent with and without each other over the years, I took a linear approach, and went down my list of days month by month. Every time I reached May, I wanted to skip over Mother's Day and go directly to the May long weekend. Not because I didn't have anything to say about Mother's Day, but because I was certain that I wouldn't like wrestling whatever I had to say into a cohesive assortment of words.

Every time I steered myself to my writing chair to tackle the topic, all my delay tactics took over. My body veered away from my desk. My dialing hand pulled me towards the telephone, certain that I had to make next year's dentist appointment at that very moment. That task complete, the nearest magazine demanded instant attention. Not a second more could pass before I read *Maclean's* cover article about whether or not I'd missed the opportunity to capitalize on the latest stock market boom. That story held my attention for no more than a few paragraphs, but my legs still would not take me to my desk. There was only one thing to do. Go outside.

On a long walk I let my mind wander, encouraged my gut to relax. Cool air made the muscles on my face alert as my brain worked to dispel my resistance. I told myself that writing about a spring event in the fall would be an invigorating experience. I began to compose an opening sentence, and then an opening paragraph for an essay on Mother's Day. But as soon as I was back inside my house, my legs took me to the kitchen, where I sat down to write out a grocery list. The next thing I knew, I was re-organizing my spice drawer. When that pressing task was finished, I stood back to admire my work, pleased to see all the jars in their new positions, arranged alphabetically from allspice to thyme. I added cinnamon to my grocery list.

List-making is sometimes a good springboard into writing. I jot down words and phrases, number them, put them in a logical order, and imagine them as an outline for something yet unknown. Sometimes even my grocery lists are quite entertaining, especially if I'm writing them for my husband, a willing grocery shopper who tends to buy what he wants instead of what I want him to buy.

Once my list was finished, I decided that the writing was messy—so messy it required redoing. This is an annoying habit of mine. My lists must be neat. If they're untidy, I lose interest in them. On a fresh sheet of paper, I printed each letter as if performing calligraphy. Below "cinnamon," I added "toilet paper," along with specific instructions that my husband was not to buy the plushy bleached stuff that's bad for the environment. Then I crumpled up the list and threw it into the recycling bin. Why risk it? I went straight to the store and bought the toilet paper myself.

I didn't want to write about Mother's Day because over the years I'd come to dislike it. My antipathy grew slowly, similar to lichen on granite or barnacles on a humpback whale. This admission will no doubt cause eyebrows to raise and foreheads to furrow, especially on the faces of other mothers. I might as well proclaim that I don't like clean air or puppies. (I like both those things.)

I eventually did get myself into my writing chair that day. At about two o'clock in the afternoon, I plunked my butt down onto the cushioned seat and opened my laptop. After I'd stretched out my hands and my wrists, my wayward fingers betrayed me as soon as they touched the keyboard. They wanted to check my e-mail, update my Facebook status, and dash off a Twitter post. At moments like that, I've learned that it's better to satisfy those urges than resist them, otherwise they get in my way, like itches that need scratching. After completing those chores, my fingers took me to YouTube, where I watched the original video of John Lennon's "Imagine" several times and wondered if I'd reached my one hundredth viewing yet. My favourite part was still when John and Yoko magically disappear through the front door of the big white house.

By this time it was three o'clock. Obviously, this particular procrastination was a stubborn one, so I had to trick it. Still on YouTube, I typed in the words "Mother's Day" and found a video of two brothers taking a picture of themselves as a present for their mother, one all dressed up, the other wearing a T-shirt with the word "TOOL" on it. The dressed-up brother insists that the Tool brother put a tie on. When the Tool brother returns with a yellow tie around his neck, he is still wearing the "TOOL" shirt. The dressed-up brother punches him, and the fight is on. Two minutes of hilarity later, at least I was thinking about Mother's Day.

But my fingers were still not trustworthy, so I decided to get away from my keyboard and start the writing process by hand. With that, my body took me off on a hunt for the perfect pencil and the ideal pad of paper. I like my "thinking" paper to be lined, otherwise my handwriting grows bigger and bigger, expanding to fill the available space until I average about three words a page.

Despite my discomfort about Mother's Day, I willingly honoured my own mother each year: not elaborately, usually with a card and a phone call, perhaps some flowers. The usual. I wasn't very original in buying her Mother's Day gifts. Maybe that was because I didn't give it much consideration. But I'd rather think that it was because my mom seemed to enjoy receiving these typical gestures on Mother's Day. They were what she expected to get.

And I knew that my own Mother's Day experiences were not to blame for my feelings about the day. Before I'd turned thirty, I'd become mother to three children. Each year I receive thoughtful, personalized Mother's Day cards from them, cards that tell me how much I mean to them and how much I inspire them, cards that make me want to weep with pride and do cartwheels across my front yard—except that I can't do physical cartwheels, so I do them in spirit.

Over the years, I've given the job of mothering much thought. So much so that I wrote a PhD dissertation about motherhood. That academic endeavour, combined with my personal experience, allows me to consider myself well-informed in my thinking about how motherhood affects women's lives.

Our world makes a big fuss about mothers, a fuss that carries weighty evaluations. When it comes to mothering, in the eyes of those watching—and there are many—adequate isn't good enough. Mothers are good, or mothers are bad. Those are the only categories. I put myself in the good category. Naturally. Who would put herself in the bad category? Too often the people who label some mothers as bad are other mothers. Mothers monitor mothers. It's the way of our world. I don't like it, but it's what happens. That had to be it, I thought. The reason I didn't like Mother's Day was because of the judgements mothers place on each other.

I can't remember much about how Mother's Day unfolded in the house I grew up in. I know we never brought breakfast to Mom in bed. That would have been silly—she wouldn't have been there. I can't ever remember my mother being in bed when I got up. Not only was she up, but her bed was already made. She made it almost as soon as she got out of it, as long as my father wasn't still in it. To this day, I do the same thing. I can't think straight if I haven't made my bed, and I certainly can't start working until it's done. It's like trying to write while I'm still in my pyjamas. It's not going to happen. I can't think when I'm not wearing underwear.

I do have vague recollections of making both Mother's Day and Father's Day cards when I was in elementary school. I also dimly recall Sunday brunches when we served Mom eggs, bacon, and toast at the table. We probably gave her a few small gifts—perhaps a new African violet for the kitchen window, or a fresh set of oven mitts. Then we made her stay in her chair while we cleaned up. But as the afternoon wore on, the sense of Mother's Day disappeared, and soon she would be in the kitchen preparing Sunday night's roast beef dinner as usual.

Father's Day was even less of an event; more like a regular Sunday, except that Dad got a new tie or a bottle of Old Spice aftershave along with his brunch.

Still, I was uneasy. I knew there had to be more to my Mother's Day consternation than mothers who judge other mothers. In the face of so much social measuring, most women have learned how to weather this type of pressure. So I looked at how Mother's Day compares to Father's Day. It seemed to me that both the Parent Days have attracted increased marketing emphasis in recent years, an emphasis I felt was a pushback, a reversion to so-called traditional roles, especially for women. I studied greeting cards looking for evidence. According to Father's Day cards, male parents are big and strong, funny and athletic. They throw baseballs and footballs. They give good advice, and are manly role models for their children.

Mother's Day cards are different. The idealization of motherhood is rampant, the greeting cards filled with flourishes and verses about how mothers are always loving and always sweet and always patient and always devoted. Each card seems to carry with it the implicit suggestion that, for women, mothering would and should be their primary purpose in life.

I was certain that was it. My discomfort rose out of that greeting-card ideal. Mother's Day both reflects and perpetuates a particular brand of mothering—someone who is selfless, all-wise, all-sacrificing, ever kind and good—an impossible standard. That mother is the only person capable of providing her children with the attention they need, so she must always be ready to put her own life aside. That mother makes me want to scream. I don't think her brand of mothering is healthy for herself or her family.

I confess that I fell short of that version of mothering, and admit to days when I wondered what my life would have been like if I hadn't had children. What would I have done with my years? Where would I have gone? I also admit to days when I was envious of the freedom my childless friends enjoyed, to days when I wanted to open the front door and scream into the empty street: "But What About Me!"

In our current culture of attachment parenting and child-centred family focus, I wonder how many young parents have days when they want to scream out those same words, but can't. Someone would call the authorities.

When my mother was alive and could still read, I'd stand in my favourite greeting-card store for a long time looking for the right card for this daughter to give her mother. I shuddered at the florid verse and overwrought descriptions. They were too much, too false. Not because their messages didn't apply. Some of them did. But my mother was too real to me. She didn't fit any of these cards. In the end, I always walked out with the simplest card I could find, one with only three words: Happy Mother's Day. I could write the rest myself.

Back when I was a new mother, my then-husband was adamant that I would not be getting a Mother's Day present from him— because I was not his mother. As our daughter was only seven months old, I knew she wasn't going shopping on her own. Thus, my expectations for my initial Mother's Day were modest. I wasn't that upset about it. A little disappointed maybe, but back then, making a big deal of a new mother's first Mother's Day wasn't the heady thing it's evolved into today.

Sometime during the week before that long-ago Sunday, I asked my husband if he liked being a father. It was a leading question, perhaps a wifely strategy on my part. I knew that his answer would be a definitive yes, to which I replied, "Well, if I wasn't a mother, you wouldn't be a father right now." A few days later, at a lazy Sunday morning brunch, I received a nice plastic watch with interchangeable red, white, and blue rims that allowed me to co-ordinate my new time-telling device with all my outfits. My husband shrugged his shoulders and grinned as I thanked him.

The red, white, and blue colour scheme of my Mother's Day watch was a nod to where it came from. Only now do I realize how appropriate it was that my first Mother's Day present was American-made, because both Mother's Day and Father's

Day were also made in the USA. Discovering this was an "Aha" moment for me. I'd always suspected that Mother's Day and Father's Day were manufactured celebrations that arose from fairly recent social moments rather than a slow evolution from ancient traditions.

Having a special day to recognize mothers does have a long pagan and religious history. Not insignificantly, the first mothers to receive these honours were goddesses. In ancient Greece, it was Rhea, goddess of motherhood and fertility. In ancient Rome, it was Cybele, a mountain goddess, mother, and protector.

Mother goddesses have been around for a long time. Early Christians found a human model to idealize: the Virgin Mary was custom-made for that role. And the sixteenth century saw the rise of a Church of England occasion called "Mothering Sunday," scheduled in February each year, partly to allow domestic servants the opportunity to visit their own mothers rather than serve high tea to their employers.

Despite these historical precedents, Mother's Day as we know it today is just over one hundred years old. Both Mother's Day and Father's Day originated in the twentieth century, in the United States. The first Mother's Day happened in 1872, organized by Julia Ward Howe, a Massachusetts social activist also known for writing "The Battle Hymn of the Republic." Howe's version of Mother's Day was all about peace. Having seen the violence of the American Civil War, she envisioned a day for women to gather together and discuss ways they could work towards a world without war.

But Howe's model didn't catch on. Mother's Day didn't really begin until 1908 when Anna Jarvis organized a Mother's Day campaign in West Virginia as a memorial for her own mother. What I like about Anna Jarvis is that she paid attention to the apostrophe in Mother's Day, insisting that it must indicate the singular possessive (Mother's) rather than the plural (Mothers') because in her mind, this day was meant to be a private celebration between a child and its mother.

That privacy didn't last long. Jarvis's Mother's Day became wildly popular. In fact, her efforts resulted in so much consumer attention for this new occasion that by the 1920s, Jarvis was unhappy with the day's capitalistic image. By the time of her death in 1948, she'd spent many years and much of her money campaigning against the maternal day of recognition she'd created.

Father's Day came about in response to Mother's Day. In 1910, in Spokane, Sonora Dodd organized a day to honour her father, a man who'd raised six children on his own after the death of his wife. But while Mother's Day became nationally recognized merely six years after Anna Jarvis's initial efforts, Father's Day wasn't officially acknowledged until the 1970s. The occasion was slow to achieve widespread acceptance, because people were suspicious of it. They resisted its opportunism, seeing it as a transparent marketing tactic launched by manufacturers of neckties and pipes: companies that hoped to increase their profits if Father's Day gained the same level of success as Mother's Day. Despite this slow public acceptance, the merchants and manufacturers persevered and eventually prevailed. Father's Day became an annual event on the calendar and a modest commercial success.

More recently, we've seen the addition of a Grandparents' Day, scheduled for the second Sunday in September. This understated celebration has so far been a marketing disappointment. Card manufacturers are no doubt pinning their hopes on an ageing population that produces more grandparents every day. Greeting cards festooned with the Grandparents' Day forget-me-not flower may be taking up more room on card display shelves any year now.

In the meantime, in the Parents' Days category, Mother's Day is the runaway winner. Every year, more cards and gifts are purchased for Mother's Day than for Father's Day. The reasons for this are unclear. Perhaps their time in the maternal womb leaves children feeling more intimately connected to Mom. Perhaps older and adult children are more comfortable expressing sentiment towards mothers. Whatever the reasons, Mother's Day continues to be a commercial bonanza. In the United States, more long-distance phone calls are placed on Mother's Day than on any other day of the year. Father's Day does have one winning statistic: more collect long-distance phone calls are placed on Father's Day than on Mother's Day.

So I decided that it was the economic frenzy around the Parent Days that disturbed me, but I also knew that the commercial idealization of motherhood wasn't the only source of my discomfort. Many—hopefully most—people are astute enough to recognize the difference between genuine emotion and obligatory sentimentality, so there had to more to it.

I have great empathy for today's new parents. They have so much more homework than my generation did. The amount of pregnancy, infant development, toddler training, feeding and vaccination, special schooling, and child psychology information available is infinite. At the same time, mother angst is off the charts. The result is that mothers are harder than ever on each other.

Choosing how to mother is fraught with social danger as parents wrestle with difficult questions. *Do I stay home with my children and abandon my career? Do I go to work outside my home and risk leaving my babies with someone else?* It's a quandary that has never been resolved to anyone's satisfaction. And it won't be until the corporate working world acknowledges that parenting is necessary work for both men and women, and makes room for that philosophy in their rigid business structures. Not for profit. For the social good. After all, it's the responsibility of society to ensure the viability of the next generation.

In considering the dilemmas facing parents these days, I began to think my disquiet about Mother's Day came from its requirement for us to be in mother mode all day. What if, I thought, instead of tying Mom to the usual rituals on Mother's Day, she was offered a total day off? Instead of making her sit through obligatory brunches and dinners, why not let her have the whole day to herself, a day to focus on the person she is in addition to being a mother? Let her go hiking, or to the library, or to the art gallery, or on a long bike ride, or spend the day watching three movies in a row, bringing her fresh bowls of popcorn whenever she runs out.

Not all mothers would opt for this, but what if it were available without repercussions, without guilt? What if a mother could actually choose a day away from her kids, instead of being feted as Mom? That was it, I thought. That was the source of my unease. On Mother's Day, mothers have to be mothers. Not only that, they have to be model mothers.

But my consternation still nagged at me. I felt that I'd missed something. I pored over my notes and went back over the words I'd written. Again and again. I took myself for another long walk. I went to the grocery store and bought more toilet paper. I did some yoga. I went back to my computer and watched more YouTube videos. And then it hit me, right in the middle of rereading my notes on the American origins of Mother's and Father's Days. I sat back and felt my discomfort evaporate. I'd figured out what had been bothering me.

Back in the early twentieth century, when our modern-day versions of the Parent Days originated with visions from Anna Jarvis and Sonora Dodd, they were modelled on a particular version of family. This was a rigid paradigm based on strictly gendered roles, and equally rigorous notions about how children should be raised.

But we live in an evolved world. Today, some children have three or four parents, while others have only one. Some children have two fathers or two mothers. Some have bedrooms in two homes. Some have parents they can't identify, biological parents from sperm banks or egg donors, parents that have no intention of ever getting involved with their offspring. Others have hands-on, caring adoptive parents or step-parents who share no genetic connection with their children, but love them no less.

Mother's Day and Father's Day are based on outdated models. So let's abandon these old icons. Let's pick a Sunday in between the two current dates—say the last Sunday in May or the first Sunday in June—and call it Parents' Day. Let's not make any rules—just set the day aside, make it a private day, like Anna Jarvis envisioned, a day to say thanks to all parents, regardless of gender, for their efforts, for the sacrifices they make every day on behalf of their children. Let's make it a day that won't induce inner guilt about falling short of perfection, of not fitting in with an artificial and impossible standard. Let's make it a day that simply recognizes parents for being as adequate as possible at a difficult and challenging task. It could be the best day of the year.

May Long is Tee Time

We need it. By May, we feel we've earned it. In eastern Canada, many know it as "Firecracker Day" or "May Two-Four." For those of us living in western Canada, it's simply "May Long." When the fifth month of the year moves past its middle point, the excitement builds:

"Can't wait for camping on May Long!"

"Opening up the cabin on May Long!"

"Stocking up on beer for May Long!"

May Long is party time, a time to bust out, the unofficial end of our seemingly endless Canadian winter, the unofficial beginning of that fickle entity we yearn for for the rest of the year: summer. As the big weekend nears, we pour outside, into our yards and our community parks, our lakes and campsites, our forests and mountains. No official menu rituals accompany May Long. Anything that can be cooked on a barbecue or a camp stove will do. Beverages are unsophisticated and often come out of an aluminum can.

Unsurprisingly, when this annual marker finally arrives, May Long's weather often confounds us with its temperamental volatility. But we will not be deterred. May Longers are nothing if not determined. The outdoors is a magnet. It draws us out from behind our closed doors and curtains. In western Canada, the May Long traditions of beef, beer, and barbecues carry on no matter the colour of the sky. But we do prefer blue.

When the May Long weather is unseasonal, many hung-over mountain campers wake up to find snow on their tents and canoes. Some lose their alcohol-induced fogginess during a chance encounter with a hungry bear fresh out of hibernation. During cold rainy May Longs, cabin-goers continue to launch their boats and jet skis, although the ensuing rides are usually brief, with passengers wearing waterproof jackets beneath their life preservers, and bucket hats tied under their chins.

For Canadians, May Long is our annual moment of optimism, an optimism sometimes disguised as foolhardiness or stubborn determination or painful revelry. Sometimes we get lucky, and May Long's weather is glorious. When this happy collusion between the elements and the occasion occurs, rural and urban Canadians all across the country emerge, pale-skinned from the interminable winter, looking up at the sky for hints of a joke. With relief, we remember that April Fool's Day was last month. This weekend is May's promise that summer will soon arrive. For the next three days, kites fly in city parks, cyclists fly along trails, kids fly on skateboards. Exuberance rules.

I don't have a lake cabin. And although I do enjoy mountains and hiking, I'm not a camper. I prefer a real bed at night, with a real bathroom nearby. These days, my children are adults with their own May Long plans. I could party all night if I wanted to. But the days when my long weekends consisted of three party nights in a row are happy, if blurry, memories.

I live with an avid gardener, so he plants all the pots, decides which calla lily goes where, and whether the potato ivy hangs from the tall blue pot or the square green one. So there's no point in me planting anything. If he doesn't like where I put it, he'll move it. So gardening does not fill my first fair-weather long weekend of the year. Thus, in this phase of my life, my May Long usually includes golf.

I've come to the realization that my life has compartments, separate rooms in the same house. I have my writing life, my family life, and my social life. Sometimes the doors between the rooms are wide open, the different parts of my life walking over the thresholds to visit the others. But I tend to keep the door to my golf life closed. I do this as a form of social sleight-of-hand. In some circles, it's distinctly uncool to admit to being a golfer. I came of age in the sixties, so above all else, I must be cool.

More than two decades have passed since I first picked up a golf club. In that time, I've learned that mentioning golf in a casual conversation elicits three distinct responses: complete indifference, a spark of interest that moves the conversation in a new direction, or an eye-roll of disdain that stops it entirely. Sports like skiing and snowboarding don't evoke the same sneer. They aren't considered boring by those who don't partake in them: extravagant, yes, but not boring. Golf is different. It has a hard time shedding its snobby old-men-wearing-bad-pants image.

For years, I've wrestled with my own conflicted relation-ship with golf, turned it over and over in my head. Perhaps I shouldn't golf, I tell myself at times, especially after a bad game. It's a time-consuming, money-sucking activity. I argue with my golf alter-ego, the stubborn enthusiast who's taken up residence in my head, the one who refuses to listen when I say, just think how much reading/writing/photography/hiking I'd get done in the summer if I didn't play golf.

I came to the game as an almost middle-aged adult. My husband was already a player when we met. Every time he left the house for the golf course, I was surprised when he disappeared for six or seven hours. I thought golf was like a racquetball game or a workout at the gym.

"What took you so long?" I'd ask after the first few times he went missing for almost an entire day.

"I went golfing," he'd answer, looking as if I'd asked him if the sky was still blue.

One day, I said I wanted to go with him and walk the golf course as he played. To his credit, he hesitated only a moment before agreeing. I felt as if I'd been given a pass into a secret society. It was a walk I remember well. I was careful to stay out of the way, but I watched every shot. At one point, I wanted to ask him why he hit his ball into the trees when the small hole with the flag in it was in the other direction. Fortunately, I didn't.

During that afternoon, I felt something. I'm not sure whether it originated in my head or my gut, but I was taken over by a strong urge to swing a golf club myself, an almost irresistible desire to know what it felt like to make contact with that small white dimpled ball. That night, I confessed my new desire to my husband. Again to his credit, he didn't race out and buy me a set of golf clubs. Instead, he bought me a series of lessons with a golf professional. A smart man, my husband. If I was about to invade his golf territory, he wanted me to know what I was doing.

In the years since, having watched people venture out onto a golf course too soon, I've come appreciate his wisdom. Learning to golf is more than grip, stance, and swing. New golfers need to learn where to walk, where to stand, when to talk, and when to keep quiet. They must learn that the game has a pace and a rhythm they need to understand, that there are moments for moving quickly, and moments for not moving at all.

Steeped in tradition and history, golf was originally intended for monarchs and nobility. Recent evidence suggests that a game resembling golf was played in China prior to the thirteenth century. Other evidence indicates that a "golf-like" game was played in the Netherlands in 1297. Despite these theories, the generally accepted history of golf acknowledges that the game as we know it came from fifteenth-century Scotland. I have lived and travelled in Scotland. Some of those golf courses look timeless, as if they're still in the fifteenth century.

Now played worldwide on large tracts of scenic land, golf has an undeniable history of sexism, racism, and classism. It has been deemed the domain of the elite and the upper-middle classes, the purview of white men on their way up in society at the expense of those less socially mobile. Also, in the era of climate change, golf has garnered criticism for being environmentally careless, forcing course superintendents everywhere to find more conservationist methods for maintaining the manicured beauty of their sites. This, at least, is a positive development.

Today's game is a complex blend of discipline, mystique and celebrity, a blend enhanced and complicated by the old customs and traditions. Golf's deeply embedded biases lurk beneath its calm polite veneer, in and around its pristine enclaves and elegant clubhouses. Some applauded when the most famous golf club in North America, Georgia's Augusta National, finally admitted its first female members in 2012. Others said it was an embarrassment that the historic move had taken so long. Both observations seem valid to me.

Golf's long story weaves through centuries of social and cultural upheavals, leaving it vulnerable to criticism. A lyric from Tom Russell's "Who's Gonna Build Your Wall" says that a white man wearing a golf shirt and carrying a cellphone is the scariest of all sights. Whenever I hear that song, I sing along with the catchy chorus and feel the dark truth of its central premise, a scathing commentary about the building of an

American wall to keep Mexican immigrants out of the southern United States. But I always trip over that golf-shirt cellphone line.

For one, I'd bet money that Russell has a cellphone somewhere in his instrumental kitbag. For another, while the stereotype no doubt fits in many cases, it also insults a lot of people who don't deserve it. I've met many good women and men who wear golf shirts, people who aren't the cold-hearted "fat-cat white developer" villains in Russell's song. Yes, those types can be found in the clubby bars common to all golf courses, but so can a lot of teachers, small business owners, community builders, and just plain ordinary people who happen to like what the game of golf offers.

It's a strange game, one of ups and downs. Golfers go through several internal cycles, both physical and emotional, during the time it takes to play eighteen holes of golf, which should be four hours, and too often isn't. I like four-hour golf. I can pace myself, plan my bathroom breaks, feed and water my body adequately, and stay involved in my game for that length of time. If it gets any longer, I lose interest, start thinking about what comes next in my day or evening, about the writing I abandoned on my desk, about the bread and lettuce I need to pick up at the grocery store on the way home.

On a warm May Long afternoon, I indulge myself and let my mind wander to the cold beer waiting for me in the clubhouse. If it's a cool May Long, I'll have a glass of crisp white wine instead. I've learned to let myself enjoy these treats without guilt. Getting older does bring some pleasures.

Golf is a game of tempo, of measured pace, steady progress, and personal stillness. Like life itself, it's an ongoing learning experience. I occasionally play the game well, and occasionally play it very badly. But no matter how I play, I always come away from the course with the sense that I've learned something. I learn about myself because the game is rife with opportunities for personal insight, especially about managing emotions. *Why were my hands shaking on that putt? Why did I put that tee shot in the water?* I learn about the people I play with because four hours on a golf course with three other players is a great revealer of character. *I was nervous about playing them, but I had no reason to be. They were totally gracious.*

My husband and I play golf courses wherever we go, often paired with a twosome we've never met. At first I was apprehensive about playing with strangers, but gradually I came to realize that no one was there to watch me. We were all there to play our own games. After putting out on the last hole of these rounds, we always extend our hands to our playing partners and say how much we enjoyed our time with them. Not once has anyone walked away from the game without shaking our hands. Most of the time, we never see those people again. Occasionally, we connect with the people we're paired with, and have after-game drinks with them. Once in a while, we even share contact information so we can arrange to play again. Golf puts people together for a few hours, and then sends them on their paths again. They may cross in the future—or not.

The patio at my home golf course has a generous view of both the first tee and the eighteenth green. When I sit there, I like to watch people beginning their games and others finishing theirs. The groups readying for their drives on the first tee are always focused on their pre-game preparations. Men in regular foursomes tend to banter back and forth as they establish their bets and pairings. They watch each other's tee shots carefully and head off down the fairway at a brisk pace, pulling their clubs behind them, each walking directly to their own balls.

Not many women golfers bet, so their pre-game prepara-tions consist of social chatter as they adjust their visors, smooth down their golf skirts, and put on their gloves. After they've all teed off, they walk down the fairway as a group, scattering only when they reach the first ball.

Most people want to walk the course if their bodies are able. At least, most middle-aged or older people. Young men prefer to ride. I'm always surprised at how many physically fit young men choose to take golf carts. I have a theory about why they do this. It's the cupholders. They need a place for their beer.

One of the best sights from my patio perch was watching two adolescent girls, sisters with wide matching smiles. They almost ran up to the first tee, their golf bags slung off their shoulders, the younger one taller than her sibling. The older one teed off first. The younger one followed, mimicking her sister's pre-shot routine almost exactly. The older one out-drove the younger one by about fifteen yards. As they walked down the fairway to their balls, I could see them involved in a lively conversation, could almost hear it: *I'll beat your drive on the next hole. As if.*

Golfers heading out to start their rounds have a gait and body language different from those coming in at the end. In the beginning, they stand tall, roll their shoulders and stretch their backs, readying their bodies for what's to come. They head down the first fairway with strong strides and their heads held high. For those walking down the last fairway at the end of their games, the anticipation has turned to acceptance. They've experienced what the golf course has offered that day. They've had their misses, felt the "rub of the green" go with or against them, and are already mentally putting their clubs away until the next time.

I once played a round of golf with my mother. Only once. It was fascinating for me to watch my non-athletic mother swing a club. She was surprisingly fluid, had good tempo, and usually sent the ball in the direction she wanted it to go, although not very far. I remember that we played on a cool overcast day, and I was wearing shorts. On every tee box, Mom asked me if I was warm enough. *Yes, Mom, I'm fine.* For the first few holes, I found her concern amusing. Then it started to chafe. I was a grown woman with grown children of my own, and my mother still thought that I couldn't dress myself properly. I didn't play well that day.

I sometimes think of my mother when I'm at my golf course. I see her in the older women who still play the game. One in particular makes me think of Mom. Not because they're anything alike, but because I wish my mother could see this woman. She's in her late eighties and still walks the course, pushing her clubs on a pull-cart. I like to watch as she finishes up her round for the day, and I always wonder how many times she's already played that week. I like how she walks the fairway at an even pace, the small Zen smile I can see under her visor. I like to watch her sink that final putt, which she often does. A one-putt is always a good way to finish a game. I've noticed that she often plays alone these days, her longtime playing partners all gone now. Alone out there, her aura is meditative, yogic. My eyes want to stay on her. My brain gives me a refrain: *Like that. When I get there, I want to be like that.*

Occasionally, people ask me why I play golf. I don't give the usual reasons, although I certainly see them as benefits. I do enjoy the fresh air, but I don't play golf for the air. For fresh air, I leave my golf clubs behind and go for a long walk in Edmonton's lush river valley. I've enjoyed the sculptured beauty of all the courses I've been lucky enough to visit, but I don't play golf for the scenery. For scenery, I go to the mountains or the desert or the ocean. And I don't play golf for exercise. For me, golf is an activity, not an exercise. In fact, I have to participate in other forms of regular exercise so that I can continue to get through a round of golf. I do enjoy the people I meet playing golf, but I don't play to socialize. When I'm on the golf course, I'm there to play. I socialize after the game. I especially don't play golf to relax. Anyone who plays golf regularly knows that it's not a relaxing game. It can as easily add stress to your life as reduce it.

I play golf because I like to swing the golf club and make contact with that little white ball. Whether the full swing of a tee shot or the fluid stroke of a short putt, I feel a tremendous rush when my club flows through the ball in such a way that the impact causes it to go exactly where I want to play my next shot from. When that happens, it's so satisfying that I can't wait to get to my ball and do it again.

I don't consider myself a "serious" golfer. In fact, I dislike that term intensely because it's so often issued as a backhanded compliment to a player who has the potential to score better than others. It's backhanded because it implies that so-called serious golf is incompatible with ordinary golf, or that golfers who play the game well, or play it the way it's intended to be played are somehow unfriendly. As a high mid-handicapper who might shoot an eighty-seven one day and a hundred the next, I consider myself a seriously friendly golfer.

To my dismay, I do tend to "crater" on the golf course. Fall apart. Can't make a good swing to save my sanity. I might have been playing well for nine or twelve holes when I suddenly feel different, like some alien power has taken over my body. Sometimes I get excited because I know I'm on my way to a good score. This is a sure-fire way for me to ensure that a series of triple bogeys are coming up. All at once, my legs will feel paralyzed, my shoulders will refuse to turn, and my arms will crash the club down onto the ball, squirting it ahead or even sideways, the distance gained maybe a scant fifty yards instead of a hundred and fifty.

And yes, I have thrown the occasional sand wedge out of a bunker in disgust. I've let the occasional blue epithet escape my lips, have looked around for something or someone else to blame for my own ineptitude. I'm not proud of any of those moments. But all golfers have or have had them. What I've learned over the years is how to recover from them, how to allow myself a few moments to feel my anger and then walk it off, let it go, not beat myself up for my failures.

In our sports-crazed society, golf has much to offer. It is not violent. When golf injuries occur, they aren't inflicted by other golfers. And golf is the only sport where a player calls penalties on her or himself, the only sport that relies on the player's integrity to enforce the game's rules, a sport that teaches players of all ages to be honest with themselves and forthcoming with their opponents.

Golf is also the only sport with a handicapping system based on each golfer's potential ability to score, a system that makes it possible for new and seasoned golfers to play together equitably, a system that makes it possible for male and female golfers to play together, to compete as partners and opponents. This handicap system and the rules of golf have reputations for being complicated. They aren't really. What they are is specific.

To play golf comfortably, golfers need to know the rules of the game. My favourite rule of golf is the first one. It says that no player shall waive or agree to waive any of the other rules of golf. That's right, I always think when I read it. And I want to add, if you do that, you're playing some other game. Golfers do that every day when they decide to play "ready" golf, meaning that anybody can hit or putt anytime. It changes the game. Nobody changes the rules of tennis. Nobody decides that any player can serve a tennis ball anytime they're ready. It would be chaos. It would no longer be tennis. That's what "ready" golf is. No longer golf. Many people will disagree with me on this. That's okay. I can handle it.

Knowing the rules allows players to assess their situations and consider their options. Knowing the rules allows room for creativity. It's like poetry. Good poets know how to write good prose, how to write long complex correct sentences that have many words. And it's that knowledge that gives them the freedom to eliminate the words they don't need.

From my perspective, the game of golf contributes positively to today's world. Professional golf associations and individual golf clubs all over the world run junior programs that not only teach youngsters how to play the game, and how to behave well on a golf course, but also how to play honestly and have consideration for their opponents.

And golf has a heart. Nowadays, virtually all professional golf tournaments have a charitable component. These events support everything from fighting breast cancer to funding local hospitals to creating programs for underprivileged children. And professional golfers don't go on strike against their own association for more money. If they want to make more money, they have to work hard at improving their game. They can't come to their field of play, coast through the game, and still go home with a paycheck. If professional golfers don't play well, they don't get paid. Effort reaps reward. I like that.

So while others are at their cabins, or planting their gardens, or camping beside cool clear creeks, I spend my May Longs on cool green fairways. If the weather has co-operated, I will already have played my first few rounds of the new season. On May Long, my next four months spread out in front of me like an enticing invitation. Come on, come out, come play with us, my golf clubs sing out to me. And so I go, when I can, each day thinking that maybe today is the one: the day I break eighty for the first time. I know that more than likely it won't be, that an under eighty round might never happen for me. But I'll never know for sure unless I try. That's another thing about golf. It's a sport I can keep getting better at, even as my years add up. I wonder what else we can get better at as we get older.

Lakes I Have Known

I thought my heart was going to stop. Bursting back to the surface, I gasped for air, but my lungs were still in shock. I tried to speak. Nothing came out except more gasps. On the deck of the houseboat I'd just jumped from, my husband, children, and friends were doubled over with laughter. It was the first weekend in June, the cloudless sky above us an azure umbrella. The air temperature was summer-warm, but this early in the season, the glacier-fed waters of Shuswap Lake were not.

I swam back to the boat, climbed up the ladder, and shook myself off. Then I jumped back in again. Everyone did. Time and time again. Afterwards, we rubbed our arms and compared goosebumps, touched each other's skin. We all tingled from the contrast of warm and cold. The feeling was delicious. Every nerve in my body was alert. We repeated this experience often during those three days. And almost twenty years later, we still talk about it.

The older me, especially my knees and lower back, appreciates the relief from supporting my body weight that water brings. But I sense that water's magnetic appeal is more than that. What is it about immersing oneself in water, in cool calm lakes, in the salty rolling tides of oceans, in steaming hot tubs, and warm scented baths? Are these merely cleansing rituals, or do we spend our lives forever seeking the comfort of the amniotic sac in which we gestated? And when immersed, does each plunge bring a personal baptism along with the visceral solace?

When I was a child, the July first holiday we know now as Canada Day was called Dominion Day. I remember a quieter, more staid celebration than today's national splash of pomp and colour, but it's possible that I simply lived in a much smaller world back then. Usually we had a barbecue in the backyard. I vaguely recall firecrackers going off in the lane behind our house, but that could be memory enhancement. What I liked best about July first was that summer had officially arrived, which meant school was out. And I knew that sometime before September's Labour Day weekend, our family would spend a few weeks at the lake. But before the lake, there would be swimming lessons.

At the public swimming pool near our Winnipeg house, I took to the breaststroke immediately. The front crawl was, and still is, more arduous work for me. Despite this, I earned all my Red Cross swimming badges. First Junior, then Senior. Each year, I had my mother sew the newest one beside the last one on the front lower hip of my baggy bathing suit. After Senior came the Bronze Medallion. I didn't think I'd ever pass the Medallion test because to do so I had to swim sixteen lengths of the pool, four of them using with my weak front crawl stroke. On top of that, I had to tread water for five minutes, no hands. But I did it. I think I wore that Bronze Medallion around my neck for months afterwards.

Never having owned a cabin, my lake experiences have always been either courtesy of rented places or the hospitality of relatives or friends. As the years passed, my annual lake time dwindled to a few days, maybe a weekend or two, only very occasionally more than that. Nevertheless, lakes are a fundamental part of my remembered life. And, out of all the lakes I have known, I have a formative lake, a mother lake that still shapes part of my being.

The two piers at Ponemah were long, narrow, and weathered. They reached out over the shallows of Lake Winnipeg, a lake so large that in many places, one side is not visible from the other. Each summer, my siblings, cousins, and I ran on those two piers, jumped off them, swam back to them, spread out our towels and lay our scrawny bodies down on their platforms. We sat on their railings, and skipped stones from their steps for hours. To us, they were ours. They existed for us to play on, around, beside, and under. We perched on the top rungs of their ladders and let bare feet dangle from their planks over the sand-filled, wave-churned waters. We gathered to them as if they had supernatural powers. And they did. They took us from the shore to the waves and back again. And in my mind, they still do.

The sandy-haired man with the warm chuckle and the constant Cuban cigar who made our time on those piers possible was our uncle, our mother's older brother. He's gone now, yet he remains. A man with no children of his own, he put his fatherly energies into his nieces and nephews. With him, we didn't feel underfoot or in the way. When he was around us, he liked us to be around him. Maybe that's why he provided that magical spot where the best summer days of our childhoods remain alive, where in some ways we still play on a sandy shore beside Manitoba's largest lake.

Less than an hour's drive from our Winnipeg home, the short journey to Ponemah felt like forever to the eager children sitting on top of each other in the back seat. Asking "are we there yet" almost as soon as we backed out of the driveway, we chanted the phrase at regular intervals until the familiar chain-link fence came into sight.

Hidden by hedges and trees, the main building and guesthouse weren't visible until we were inside the gate. More estate than cottage, the property was situated on several acres of land, and required a gardener. His name was Nick. Back then I thought he was ancient. In retrospect, he was probably about forty. A skinny man who always wore a battered baseball cap perched high on the back of his head, Nick had deep crevices in his craggy face, and was never without a pair of work gloves on his hands. He was gruff, but it was a friendly gruff, the kind where "you kids stay out of the tool shed" was followed by "have you kids seen the robin's nest in the north corner?"

No one slept in at the lake. On weekday mornings, we'd often wake up to the sounds of Nick's lawnmower, chainsaw, or hedge trimmer. On Sunday mornings, we'd hear the wail of bagpipes wafting over from the cottage next door, where the neighbour practiced his piping, pacing back and forth on his veranda. My parents grumbled over their morning coffees—couldn't John at least wait until noon before blowing hot air into that thing? We didn't mind at all. We'd been up for hours.

Summers in southern Manitoba are typically hot and humid, so the only clothes we needed during the day were bathing suits. We wore them in the mornings as we ate our cereal. We wore them at lunch as we ran through the house, grabbing at sandwiches. We wore them to play badminton on the croquet lawn and croquet on the badminton lawn. We wore them as we burst out of the gate, towels flung over our shoulders, hell-bent for the piers.

In the mornings, we looked after ourselves at the beach. That's what the swimming lessons back in the city were for. In the afternoons, Mom came down for a few hours. She'd swim back and forth between the piers, first a smooth breaststroke, and then a gliding sidestroke, followed by a graceful slow-motion front crawl. She always wore a white bathing cap with a big rubber flower on it. I think it was red, but it could have been yellow. I remember the day our bagpipe-playing neighbour launched a borrowed boat and took all the adults waterskiing. We watched from the piers as my mother tried to get up on the skis over and over again. The one time she did stand up, the boat stalled and she sank right back down again. The next day, her thighs were black and blue.

The piers were exactly the same length, identical twin arms reaching ram-rod straight out from the shore. At their ends, the water wasn't deep, a fact we rediscovered each year on our first dive into the lake. Fortunately, the bottom was sand, and it only took that one dive to remind us to have our arms stretched out over our heads as we launched ourselves into the water.

Day after day, we raced each other down the piers. Day after day, we ran from one to the other and back again. We did cannonball leaps from the railings. I mimicked my mother and swam between the two, practicing my swimming skills. I didn't do the front crawl nearly as much as the other strokes. From a young age, I knew this about myself—I practice what I like to do, and resist practicing what I don't.

As the sun descended lower in the late afternoon sky, we had to be dragged away from our piers to get cleaned up for dinner. Most evenings we spent playing cards or doing jigsaw puzzles in the guesthouse because our parents wouldn't allow us to go down to the beach after dinner. Sometimes, my oldest cousin and I snuck out the guesthouse's bathroom window. We'd sit on the rocks staring at the water. If the wind was up on the big shallow lake, the rocks got wet, and so did we.

Ponemah is so close to Winnipeg that it's possible to work a full day in the city and drive out for the night. My father did this often. Occasionally, he brought guests back with him. One day, Mom prepared us with her usual speech. Dad was bringing a business associate out for the night, and we were to be on our best behaviour.

My father was not a small man, about 5'10" with a sturdy build. That evening, when he and his guest walked in, I couldn't help staring. Dad looked puny. His friend's belt seemed to be at the same level as my father's shoulders.

Dad beckoned us over. "Say hello to Mr. Markham, kids. He's visiting from Ontario." We looked up, way up, and mumbled hello.

The giant smiled down. "I'm mighty glad to meet you all."

And it was done. He would forever be Mighty Markham.

While my mother prepared supper, the men decided to go for a swim. On hearing this, four siblings and two cousins looked at each other in dismay. A few minutes later, as Dad and Mighty Markham strolled down one pier's narrow wooden planks, six worried children stood peering through the chain-link gate, watching every step they took. Even from our confinement in the yard, we were certain we could hear the pier groaning, creaking, agonizing. We could see the sway as each section laboured under every Mighty Markham footfall. When he dove into the water, our eyes fixed on the pier's legs. We wanted to see if the level of the lake went up with him in it.

That evening, we watched every move Mighty Markham made. In the morning after he left, we wondered if the springs on his bed had survived. So we jumped on it, all six of us at the same time.

We never saw him again. Years later, my father told me that Mr. Markham had really enjoyed his evening at Ponemah, that the band of kids shadowing him and breaking into suppressed fits of laughter every time he moved did not offend him. He wouldn't allow my parents to reprimand us, saying that he was used to comments about his size. After all, we were only kids.

Towards the end of August, with the summer days growing shorter and the waves crashing higher and louder around the thin legs of our piers, I'd stand at the beach bundled in my warmest sweater, and wonder what they looked like smothered in snow. I worried about them. How would they survive the ice floes and punishing cold? I feared they'd be gone when we returned next summer. But they never were. They were always there, the brown muddy water still lapping at those skinny wooden supports.

I don't remember consciously deciding not to go to Ponemah anymore. Growing up just got in the way. By the time I was fifteen, I had a summer job in the city. After a season or two of watching the summer place sit empty much of the time, my uncle put it up for sale. Before we realized what was happening, it was gone.

On a recent trip to Winnipeg, I rented a car and drove out to the lake. I didn't need a map. My memory took me directly there. I parked on the same grassy spot near the old garage. Once out of the car, I inhaled the reedy sea air, not salty but marine-like nevertheless. Lake air.

At the shore, the water was high and the beach submerged. Only one pier remained. I walked out along its wooden planks and leaned over the railing at the end. After a few minutes, I made a slow turn, knowing that from there I'd have a clear view of our old place. It looked different, was now painted an unfamiliar light grey. But when I closed my eyes, it was the warm dark brown colour I remembered, and two piers still reigned at Ponemah.

I knew other lakes as a child. A few times, we were invited for a weekend with some friends of my parents. Mom and Dad instructed us to call them aunt and uncle, even though we weren't related to them. Every time I did this, it felt fake to me, and even though I liked them a lot, I started thinking of them as my fake aunt and uncle. Like my parents, they had a bunch of kids and a dog. Like my father, my fake uncle was gregarious and had a taste for rye whiskey. Their cottage, an intimate informal structure with many little bedrooms, was at Falcon Lake. Located in eastern Manitoba's Whiteshell Provincial Park, it was, and probably still is, a clear, rock-bottomed lake. It had no piers. Falcon Lake had docks. Piers are high and narrow, designed to carry people over rough shallow waters out to swimming depths. Docks are short and sturdy, lower to the water, designed for mooring boats and relaxing in lawn chairs. During one memorable weekend at Falcon Lake, three things happened. I think I was twelve at the time. Maybe eleven. Possibly thirteen.

Looking for a place to change into my bathing suit, I burst into a bedroom and saw my fake uncle naked. He was the first naked adult male I'd ever seen. I didn't say a word, just stood there, staring. He didn't react at all, simply asked me if I was having a good time as he pulled on his swimming trunks. I never told anyone, especially not my mother. She would have been mortified.

I dove off the dock and swam for a long time. I swam out into the lake as far as I dared, until I got nervous that a motorboat might run over me. I swam all the way back to shore, past the dock to the rocks at the end. I tried to walk on them, but they were wet and slimy, so I swam to the end of the dock and climbed up the ladder. Wrapped in a big towel, I stood shivering in the middle of the lawn chairs, all occupied by adults having their cocktails. Someone said my lips were blue. I looked down and saw what I thought was a leaf on my foot. I tried to brush it off, but it didn't budge. It felt slimy and cool to the touch. "That's a bloodsucker," said my fake uncle.

I was unfamiliar with leeches because my formative lake, Lake Winnipeg, with its sandy bottom and roiling waters, did not have them. The thought of some creature sucking my blood hijacked my normally sensible self. I started hopping around the dock, screaming "Get it off! Get it off!" My fake uncle reached down and swiped it off my foot. My fake aunt said that wasn't a good thing to do. "You're supposed to put salt on it, Bill."

Later that afternoon, a huge storm blew in. The wind was so strong that at one point, all the children cowered under the big dining table inside the cottage, our mothers hovering nearby. My father and my fake uncle stood at the window watching the sky, discussing whether the boat would stay attached to the dock.

In its wake, the storm left fallen trees criss-crossing the driveway, their tips and branches tangled together so that they formed a tent over the vehicles. Not one dent showed on any of the cars. For many decades, in my mind, that was the biggest storm I'd ever been in. I can still hear that wind.

I'd probably experienced the same amount of wind in a Manitoba blizzard or two, but somehow we feel more prepared for those. We hunker down and stay inside. If we have to go out, we don our armour of parkas and toques. Without those things, we feel frailer. Summer storms strike when we're wearing flip-flops and tank tops. They render us vulnerable and leave us with a sense of betrayal. It's just not fair, I often hear people say after a sudden summer storm has turned a day of fun into a rush for cover. A man I was once married to had a pragmatic way of looking at events like unpredictable, unfair storms: life isn't full of round corners, he'd say, and no one ever promised life would be fair.

One summer, my husband and I drove from Alberta to Ontario's Lake of the Woods. I say Ontario because we went to an Ontario part of the lake. This enormous lake also spreads into Manitoba and Minnesota. This wasn't my first time at Lake of the Woods, but I hadn't been there for many years. I have blurry memories of going to an Anglican church summer camp on one of its fourteen thousand islands when I was about twelve, or maybe thirteen. I slept on a claustrophobic bottom bunk, swam out to the raft in the small bay, and developed a crush on one of the counsellors. Besides those three murky images, the only memories of church camp I have are of the huge lake's tall pine trees, the many channels between islands, and the birds. Winnipeg had a lot of birds, but none of them were this big. I saw my first bald eagle at Lake of the Woods.

Years later, the lake looked the same to me. We passed island after island as my uncle ferried us from Keewatin to the small dot of land where he and my aunt, my mother's sister, had built a summer cottage. For the next few days, we enjoyed a classic lake weekend. My son caught his first fish. My two daughters fell in love with an old English sheepdog named Ralph. And we watched my mom and her sister float in the lake. A few body lengths off the end of the dock, they lay on the lake surface without effort, without movement, their hands and toes visible above the water, chatting as if they were sitting at the kitchen table.

My children were fascinated by the sight. As my daughter would say years later at her grandmother's funeral, it was like watching magic happen. I was also fascinated and a little unsettled. I couldn't remember ever seeing my mother float like that. How had I become an adult without knowing that she could stay on top of water as if suspended from the sky, without any support from below, without moving her hands and feet to keep herself up? How many other things about my mother didn't I know?

The prominent lake of my adult years is in British Columbia. The amount of time I've spent there has not been considerable, but it has been memorable. For several years, we had family gatherings at a rented place on the west shore of Okanagan Lake, a large, deep body of water that is strikingly beautiful. Almost every day, its surrounding hills go through every shade of purple and blue at both dawn and dusk.

I remember the last time my mother was at Okanagan Lake, perhaps the last time she was at any lake. We all piled into our rented boat and cruised out to the middle. It's our favourite thing to do. Find a good spot without much boat traffic around, and shut the motor off. Then we throw colourful foam noodles into the water and jump in after them. We float around, get back in the boat, and jump in the water again. One afternoon, we managed to convince Mom to come with us. In her mid-seventies by now, she hesitated at first, until we reminded her that she liked riding in boats, she just didn't like skiing behind them.

Out in the middle of the lake, the water was calm. We convinced Mom to jump in, and she did. Well, she didn't really jump. She slid gently off the boat's swim deck and entered the water with barely a splash. And there she was, floating in a lake again, this time with the help of a noodle, the smile on her face Mona Lisa-like. She needed a little help getting back into the boat, but her sons-in-law were up to the task. She wore her Mona Lisa smile for the whole boat ride back to the cottage. Afterwards, she didn't say much, just that the lake had felt good, oh so good.

Nowadays when I'm immersed in the waters of a lake or a sea or even a swimming pool, I lie back and float like my mother did, my hands and feet out of the water. I don't remember being able to do this earlier in my life. Maybe it's an ageing thing, maybe our bones get lighter as we get older, maybe their porosity allows us to float without effort at this particular stage of life. Maybe we lose it again as we go from newly senior to elderly, from having confidence in our bodies to wondering if today is the day they're going to present us with the ultimate betrayal.

When I float, I like to let the water come up over my ears so I can't hear anything. I like the feeling of my hair sifting out sideways from my head. The purpose is to lose my land bearings, so I stare at the sky and let myself go. I don't sink, I drift where the wind or current takes me. And that's what it is about water. Pure freedom. Until I bump into something.

Cornucopia Soup

In the family I came from, our Thanksgiving dinner was always a traditional turkey meal. We needed a large turkey, usually about twenty-five pounds, so our bird required a lot of cooking, a whole day of cooking, from about eight o'clock in the morning onwards. I'd be up early, breaking bread for the stuffing while Mom fried the onions, celery, and sausage meat. As my brother and sisters got older, they'd help too. Sometimes we ate more bread than we put in the big metal bowl, and Mom would have to send Dad to the nearest grocery store for another loaf. When we had enough broken bread, we'd start peeling potatoes, lots of potatoes. At suppertime, the burnished brown turkey came to the table on a big platter, and Dad carved it in front of us, sharpening a long carving knife on a honing rod with great flourish before slicing into the juicy bird.

When Dad found the wishbone in the carcass, he'd put to the side of the meat platter. After dinner, during cleanup, Mom would hang it in the window over the kitchen sink. For the next several days, we'd all watch that bone wither and pale. When it was brittle enough, we'd argue about which lucky two kids got to break it. The two breakers would each make a wish. The one who ended up the biggest piece of broken bone was the winner, whose wish was then supposed to come true. We never said our wishes out loud, and I don't remember what any of my wishes were.

On the day after Thanksgiving, I think my mother made soup from all those turkey bones. I hope she did. I wish I could remember for certain, but I can't.

In the family I created, we've never carved the turkey at the Thanksgiving dinner table. We've done everything else my birth family did, with my children taking the bread-breaking roles, and me frying the onions and celery. As an occasional vegetarian, I eliminated the sausage meat from my stuffing recipe early on in my turkey-cooking career. But other than that, I've modelled our Thanksgiving dinner on the ones my mother made, except that my husband carves the turkey in the kitchen, usually with all of us standing around watching. Then we carry the heavy platter piled with steaming sliced meat to the table, where we pass it around, each one balancing the big plate as her or his neighbour takes a helping.

Before diving into our loaded plates, we say a word of thanks. Grace. My mother-in-law is usually with us. Her presence ensures that the grace is a real prayer, not my dad's old adage of "Good food, good meat, good God, let's eat," or my brother's "Rub-a-dub-dub, thanks for the grub," the ones that always made my mother shake her head at them both.

The day after a turkey dinner, I make soup. Almost always.

Widespread social attitudes towards loneliness and lonely people aren't pretty. They go something like this: It's your own fault: lonely people are weak; normal people don't feel this way; you should fix your personality defect. But loneliness is not some kind of dissonance or character flaw. It's also not uncommon. And because the condition is exacerbated by social attitudes, it becomes a silent suffering. Lonely people, should they admit their situation to themselves, tend to absorb those attitudes: *I can't let anyone know I'm lonely, otherwise people will think there's something wrong with me.* It's a nasty circle. People see unsmiling loners, not their loneliness. And the lonely deny their loneliness rather than trying to understand it. Eventually it becomes chronic, challenges their health, and evolves into a disorder.

As a theme, loneliness resists genre, location, and time. Loneliness exists in politics, nationality, religion, families, art, dance, literature. Think of Mary Shelley's *Frankenstein* and the crushing solitary world of her monster. Think of Alfred Lord Tennyson's "The Lady of Shalott," floating on her barge down that meandering river, hand trailing in the water in her drift to death.

Music is full of loneliness: The Beatles' "All the Lonely People," Roy Orbison's "Only the Lonely," Hank Williams' "I'm So Lonesome I Could Cry." Almost any Hollywood movie has a lonely theme or sub-theme: *Taxi Driver*, *Edward Scissorhands*, *American Beauty*, *Forrest Gump*, *Lost in Translation*, *The Big Chill*, *Sideways*, *Psycho*, *Silver Linings Playbook*. And those are just my favourites. Television is filled with lonely characters: Homer Simpson, Charlie Harper, Dr. House, Dexter, Don Draper, Betty Draper. Heck, any of the *Mad Men* characters.

Loneliness is all around us. It's a fundamental element in our entertainment world. We watch it, read about it, listen to it. We connect to it. But we don't want to admit that we feel it ourselves. And I think we all do at one time or another. Married people in stable relationships can be lonely. People can be surrounded by many others and still feel lonely.

I've sometimes wondered if lonely extroverts are lonelier than lonely introverts, who have learned how to distinguish between loneliness and solitude, how to save themselves from the former and seek out the latter when needed. Loneliness can happen to entire groups or communities. Loneliness is a condition of starvation, an absence of connection, a malnourishment of the psyche. A lack of soup.

I make a lot of soup in November. It's a brown month for me. Well, not completely. My twins were born in November, and that event is one of the best things that ever happened in my life. But other than their birthday, November is a sombre month of overcast skies and barren woods. My mood is often the same colour as the bark on those leafless trees. It's a month for hunkering down, for contemplation, for remembering history. On the eleventh day of the eleventh month, as I pin two poppies onto my coat, one red and one white, I wish for the tetra-billionth time that our stupid world would finally give up on the idiocy of war. If I were inclined towards depression, November would be my worst month.

I've always thought of myself as a calm person, not swayed too much one way or the other by troublesome emotions. If something I wished for didn't work out, I'd find something else. Malleable, that's me. Some may say a little dissociative, but I prefer malleable. Flexible, able to bend with the circumstances and situations life has thrown my way. Maybe it's a lack. Perhaps we're born with a finite amount of emotion to use up in our lifetimes. Maybe I was too calm in my younger years, and didn't spend enough of my lifetime emotional quotient. Maybe that's why I feel so much now. Or maybe we feel more as we get older, feel it while we can.

As the Leo-born, eldest child in a big noisy family, I'd always assumed that I was an extrovert. Our world loves extroverts. People who walk into a room and make it their own, people who gravitate towards people, who not only shine in crowds, but seek crowds they can shine in. As the mother of a medium-sized noisy family, I sometimes sought the privacy of a quiet space. When my children were still living at home but no longer in need of my constant attention, I sometimes stole away to watch a matinee movie in an almost-empty theatre. Regardless of the movie's quality, it was the time alone I relished. I began to realize that I wasn't a genuine extrovert. I was comfortable in my own company and often uncomfortable at parties, where I hovered around the edges, watching my husband flit effortlessly from group to group while I just wanted to go home.

What I didn't realize at the time was that I still had much company in my daily life; that a teenager watching television in the family room while I was sitting in my reading chair in the next room was company. I didn't realize that sitting in the same chair reading with no one watching television in the next room would feel different. I was home alone. I didn't realize that a time might come when my own company wasn't so comfortable.

My husband and I used to tell our kids that by the time they reached the age of twenty-five, we expected them to be living elsewhere. It's not that we didn't love them. It's that they had their lives to live, and we had ours. As we waited for all three to reach the declared age, we planned how we'd renovate our house (yet again) to change it into a two-person haven. But when the last of our young adults moved out for good, a little past the age of twenty-five but not yet twenty-six, we did nothing to the house. We'd lost the motivation. It didn't feel like a two-person haven. It felt both cluttered and empty.

Fast-forward a few years. After decades of paid employment topped off by eight years as a contract instructor of university-level English, I decided to pursue a full-time writing career. I looked forward to spend my days writing, to sending out my work to publishers, to seeing it published. It sounds so simple. And so I sat at home and wrote. I sat at home and ate. I sat at home and read. I sat at home and looked out the window. My daily routine rotated inward. I avoided social contact. I didn't go to movies by myself anymore. I no longer wanted to cook big family dinners. My relished solitude gradually evolved into a deeply entrenched loneliness. I craved soup much of the time.

I make all kinds of soup. I might do it on any day of the year, in any season, but my most intense soup-making season is autumn. My favourite soup-making day is the one after a turkey dinner. If it's not the day after a turkey dinner, I might create an earthy mushroom broth. But the soup I make most often is chicken. When I make it in the fall, I call it flu season soup. For several days, I immerse myself in a process that results in a steaming savoury pot filled to its brim. Real soup from real food. Soup that requires no can opener. Medicine in a bowl.

Soup-making is self-prescribed therapy for me. When I need to distract myself from something in my life, like my empty house, or the feeling that I should call my mother; when I need to work something out in my head, like a difficult conversation I should initiate but don't want to; or when a malaise creeps over me that I can't seem to shake; I make soup.

The first step in my process is to go to the market. I am in search of a whole chicken—a happy, unfettered, free-ranging, ground-pecking, clucking-at-will-into-the-barnyard-air chicken. I share a few obligatory weather-related observations with the market vendor, generally about the amount of snow we already have on the ground, what day the snow will finally arrive, or how long the snow will last this winter. As I pick through the vendor's chicken bin, I will reject one because it's too small, and another because it's lopsided. Finally my hand will fall on a bird that feels right, feels like a happy, calm (albeit dead) chicken. I like the ones with plump thighs and a balanced shape. I don't know why that matters, but it does. I definitely don't let myself think about how much happier my chicken would be if it weren't destined for my soup pot.

With my chosen fowl in my basket, I stroll around the market gathering the rest of my ingredients: onions, carrots, celery, and fresh herbs. Whatever looks perky. Nothing wilted goes into my soup.

Many years ago, when I trained as an X-ray technician, I studied anatomy. X-ray training made my nineteen-year-old brain come alive in new ways. The bored girl who survived high-school Physics with a barely passing grade of fifty-two per cent had become a thirsty sponge. Once into my training as a radiographer—that's the more professional-sounding name for an X-ray technician—I aced my Physics course. That information did not stick; now I can't remember any of it.

Anatomy class was different. What I learned there must have welded itself to the marrows of my body. Those corporeal nouns and adjectives still come easily onto my tongue: zygoma, patella, metatarsal, mandible, sphenoid, fibula. I like saying them out loud. Especially when I'm alone in a large room with high ceilings, where the words can echo around and bump into each other.

During our X-ray training, all students had to watch an autopsy. I was dreading it, but also damn curious. A senior student told me to put some gum in my pocket before going to the morgue. She didn't say why.

In our pristine white lab coats, my peers and I filed down a long hospital hallway. The further down the hall we got, the quieter it was. It didn't sound like part of the hospital at all. At the end of the hall, we entered a room, all clean and green and polished, not a soft surface anywhere—hard floor, hard ceiling, hard light. We stood in a semi-circle around a table. A body lay under a sheet. A doctor fiddled with his tools. The first thing I noticed was that the doctor wasn't wearing a mask. And neither were we. I'd been in the operating theatres, where everyone was gowned and masked, on guard against invisible threats entering the room. Sterility wasn't an issue here.

I could have used a mask. The most overwhelming part of the experience was the smell, a mixture of formaldehyde and decay so pungent that I felt as if I could reach into the air and touch it. As soon as it hit my nostrils, I knew what the gum was for. Some of my peers had to retreat during the procedure, but I remained on my feet all the way through that autopsy by chomping on my cinnamon-flavoured Dentyne. Strangely enough, that's my most vivid memory of that experience: the smell and the gum. I know I watched the whole procedure, but my brain refuses to remind me what I saw.

Back home from the market, I wash all the veggies. Nothing dirty goes into my soup. Then I chop onions. As the moist white pile grows on my cutting board, I chop and cry, cry and chop. I wipe my face on my sleeve, then chop and cry some more. I shake my knife at the ceiling and the grey sky outside my window, then continue to cry and chop. During this whole process, I am careful to avoid my fingers. Blood definitely does not go into this soup.

When the pile of onions spills off the cutting board onto the counter, I stop. This is usually when I pour myself a glass of wine. White. Always cold white. Even in winter. I don't know why, and I don't ask myself why. I just pour. After one long sip that I roll around in my mouth, I add three cubes of ice to my glass. Then I chop the carrots, celery, and all the herbs without shedding any tears at all.

It's often at this point that I realize I'm missing an ingredient. Sometimes it's garlic, so I'll search my refrigerator's crisper bins all the way through the top layers to the bottom. I always find some. I'll pull off two cloves and peel them. But they usually look too puny for the big pot, so what the heck, I peel the whole head. If I make the mistake of licking my fingers at this point, my iced white wine is at the ready.

A human being left alone for long enough will die. We need contact with each other, both physical and emotional contact. People were not meant to be completely alone. That's why solitary confinement has long been used as punishment in prisons. That's why exile and banishment and shunning have long been used as forms of behavioural control. Conform to social and cultural expectations, or suffer the lonely consequences.

Unlike love or joy, sorrow or despair, loneliness is not an emotion, although its presence evokes emotion. Loneliness is a condition, one created by external circumstances, either chosen or imposed. Some loneliness is momentary or transitional, a temporary situation remedied sooner rather than later. More serious is chronic loneliness, a state that continues for a long period of time, years, even decades, perhaps whole lifetimes, a state that results in disconnection and worse.

I've read that symptoms of loneliness include sleep disorders, high blood pressure, depression, restlessness, a head full of noise, and appetite changes. Lonely hearts beat slower. Lonely people are anxious, distracted, and have sluggish reactions to stress. In extreme cases, a lonely person goes from consuming complex books to reading only simple paragraphs without anyone noticing. Then one day you take your mother out for lunch, and realize that she can no longer read a menu. Long-term loneliness can lead to dementia. I've also read that acting to escape loneliness may result in rash behaviour, impulsive

relationships, and poor judgement. Not acting to escape loneliness may result in dementia.

Cornucopia is one of my favourite words, along with all
my anatomy words (and select others such as "myriad" and
"cacophony"). But cornucopia is special. Like viscerality, I
like the way its syllables roll off my tongue. I like the way my
lips have to make five different shapes to say it: round, pursed,
round again—more intense this time—then pressed lips to spit
out the "pee," which leads to the releasing finale of the fly-away
"ah." Cor-new-coh-pee-ah. It's like a breathing exercise, a yogic
exhalation.

A cornucopia horn resembles the top end of a tuba without
the flared part. Normally depicted lying on its side like a conch
shell, the horn is usually made out of woven plant material,
unless the maker was a sculptor with a welding shop, in which
case it might be constructed from metal tubing or old cutlery.
Plenty spills out of a cornucopia. The plenty can be grapes,
tomatoes, onions, or eggplant. Again, if the horn came from
a welder, the plenty might be nuts, nails, wrenches, or small
iconic skulls.

As a child, from my pre-kindergarten years until well into
elementary school, I coloured a paper outline of a cornucopia
almost every October. This exercise required the use of almost
all the waxy sticks in the crayon box—several shades of brown
for the woven basket with its curvy tail, orange for the pumpkins scattered around it, red for the tomatoes, yellow for the
gourds and onions, deep purple for the eggplant, and green for
the, well, greenery.

Back then, I thought Thanksgiving was a boring holiday. No presents. No chocolate eggs. No Christmas tree. No
excitement. Just a turkey dinner on Sunday evening, and a
day off school on Monday. I usually spent both days reading,

except when I had to help Mom prepare food or watch over my siblings. Sometimes Dad put me to work outside raking leaves. I liked raking leaves, and often popped a chunk of salted raw potato into my mouth on my way through the kitchen out to the backyard. Still, Thanksgiving didn't rank high on my special occasions list.

Now Thanksgiving is one of my favourite holidays. The fresh fall air. The vibrant leaves. I especially like the timing of our Canadian Thanksgiving, the second Monday in October. With our shorter growing season, it makes sense to have it earlier than the American celebration in late November. Our October date makes Thanksgiving truly a harvest holiday, one that is still far away enough from Christmas that we don't feel those pressures yet. The warm days of August and the brilliant ones of September are still fresh in our minds.

Emotionally, I find Thanksgiving the calmest of the big annual holidays. I've grown to savour its low-key commercial fuss, its lack of gifty expectations, its uncomplicated food traditions. I relish the relaxed buildup to the day, although that certainly identifies me as a city-dweller. The weeks leading up to Thanksgiving may not be so relaxed out in farm country, where harvesters are rushing to beat early frosts.

I enjoy a simple recipe for a successful Thanksgiving. Shop for good food and prepare it well, I sometimes say to myself as I'm shopping and preparing. For decorations, simply scatter a few yellow gourds down the centre of the table. Sometimes we have twelve people sit down for Thanksgiving dinner in our house. Sometimes it's thirteen, which means that two people have to sit together at one end. That's fine, because not only can our table grow quite long, it's also wide. And I have no aversion to the number thirteen.

In recent years, after my husband took some cooking lessons from a chef and learned how to debone a turkey, our

Thanksgiving dinner routine changed a little. Now we do all the work the night before. My husband dissects the turkey and arranges the breasts, drumsticks, and thighs in a roasting pan. I collect the remaining bones, skin, sinew, and scraps to make the soup stock. While the stock bubbles on the stove, we break the bread and make the stuffing, which must be cooked in a foil-wrapped baking dish because there is no turkey cavity left to stuff it into. The next morning we sleep late because a deboned turkey needs to cook for only a few hours. It doesn't have to go into the oven until mid-afternoon. We're usually up by then.

When October comes around, and I begin to stock our house for Thanksgiving, I occasionally think about how far our menu has expanded beyond my mother's. These days, our Thanksgiving dinners are a bit of a mash-up. Along with the deboned turkey, the baked-in-the-oven dressing, the mashed potatoes, gravy, peas, and Brussels sprouts (my husband feels we can simplify our menu by eliminating these), we also have some mushroom tempeh, or a quinoa salad, and maybe an Asian noodle dish. This is to satisfy the semi-vegan, fully vegetarian, and flexitarian diners that, to our great joy, now populate our lives.

Still, the next day, I make soup. Almost always.

I keep my stockpot in the lowest, darkest, most-awkward cupboard in our kitchen. When I pull it out, the first thing I do is blow the dust off its lid, whether it's dusty or not. I blow out of habit, because my mother taught me that anything stored in a cupboard might have dust on it.

I apologize to the once-happy, now dead chicken as I rinse it under the tap, shake it dry, and peer into its rear end. I don't know what I'm looking for, so I'm not sure why I do this. I just do. Several times. Then the chicken goes into the stockpot on top of all the chopped veggies, followed by a few additional ingredients: a handful of peppercorns, a palmful of sea salt, a fistful of dried bay leaves, and cool fresh water to cover it all.

My pots all have glass lids because I like to see what's going on inside them. With the heat on high, I stand watching until the water comes to a boil. And yes, my watched pot does eventually boil. I find that sighing deeply as I wait helps speed up this part. When the surface of the water resembles a hot tub with its jets on high, I turn down the heat and watch the bubbles settle to a simmer. I'm looking for an unaggressive simmer—a friendly, yet assertive bubbling. The once-happy dead chicken must be tender-cooked, not boiled to a second death. Heat level established, I set the timer for one hour and head for the couch.

Sometimes I'm not too sure how long the timer has been beeping when I roll off the couch and head back to the kitchen. Off goes the element, off comes the pot from the stove. I take the still-whole chicken out of the pot by stabbing it with two serving forks. I raise it slowly, dripping a trail of hot broth as I transfer it to a cutting board. It's dissection time—hot and icky, but fun. I rip the drumsticks from the carcass and peel the skin back from the breasts. The whole thing ends up in gleaming juicy pieces, some sliding off the cutting board onto the counter.

Good tender chunks of meat go into a clean bowl. Skin, bones, and other remnants all go back into the stockpot. I say ouch a lot because the chicken is hot. And slippery. When I'm finished, I cover the good meat bowl and put it into the refrigerator but only after I've tasted a few of the most succulent pieces.

Then I add two glugs of cider vinegar to the pot and return it to the stove. This time I set the heat to a slightly higher level. A more aggressive simmer is fine now because the chicken is not only dead, it's in pieces. I set the timer for another hour and make a pot of herbal tea. Settling back into my recliner chair, I savour a few warming sips. The next thing I hear is an insistent dinging sound.

Once the stock has cooled down enough that it won't burn my skin if it splatters, I pour it from the pot through a colander into a large metal bowl. All the soggy solids caught in the colander go into the garbage, because all the nutrients have been cooked out of them, and they're no good for composting because they have animal fat in them. I take the garbage out to the back lane immediately after putting this sodden hodgepodge into it. If I don't, I'll regret it the next morning when I come downstairs and smell it before I step into the puddle on the floor.

The big bowl of fresh stock goes into the fridge overnight. If the fridge is full, it goes into the barbecue (not in use, of course) on our back deck, because where I live, autumn nights are as cool or cooler than refrigerator temperature, but not quite cold enough to freeze a huge bowl of liquid in ten hours.

Loneliness feels like a hole somewhere in the body, somewhere between the neck and the legs. Sometimes the hole aches so much that the pain radiates down the legs and the arms. Where loneliness isn't felt is in the head. It's a body pain. In the head, it's subject to rationalization. The introvert says I choose to be alone; I'm better off alone; the wonderful silence lets me think; I can breathe when I'm alone. The extrovert stands in the middle of a throng of familiar people wondering why the high isn't there anymore. And wanders off to find new people.

The prevailing notion is that all introverts are lonely, and that all lonely people are shy introverts. Neither is the case. Introverts are not necessarily lonely, and are often not shy at all. Many introverts are good public speakers, comfortable addressing a crowd. The successful introvert can be as well-adjusted, and perhaps even more so, than the glorious shining extrovert who takes every room as his or her own upon entering. I suspect that the extrovert suddenly left alone will skip the serenity of solitude and get to loneliness much sooner that the introvert.

Most introverts understand loneliness very well because they've had to save themselves from chronic loneliness by achieving a balance between their aversion to mingling with people and their need for solitude. They also understand that too much solitude leads to severe disconnection. It spins out of control and results in alienation. Our society mistrusts introverts because they seem to prefer aloneness. We want the world to be populated with shining, glorious extroverts. Now that would be a noisy world. Would anyone ever hear what anyone else said?

I've come to the conclusion that I'm an introvert with strong extrovert tendencies. Or vice versa. Or perhaps I'm an introvert one day, and an extrovert the next. Or perhaps I don't care anymore. Labels are restrictive and of decreasing interest to me. More useful is knowing that I don't even want to be near me when I've had no downtime. I get cranky and snappish. When I've had too much downtime, I have trouble moving myself through leaden air and become prickly with those around me.

That's when I know that my solitude has thickened and turned to loneliness. When my chats to invisible people who aren't in the room with me fall silent, I have to acknowledge that I've run out of ghosts to converse with. That's when I know it's time to put my feet into some shoes—any shoes, this is no time to get picky, that's a stall tactic—walk out the door and put myself in a situation where I'm around real people. I musn't let myself overthink it, just go to a place that has people, maybe a swimming pool where I can do laps, keeping my eyes open so I can see the legs and arms of other people in the lanes beside me. Or a coffee shop. I'll take a book to read or writing to work on, but I look up often at the people around me. Are they in groups? Pairs? Do I see anyone alone? Is what they are doing any different from what the others are doing?

The next morning, I skim the congealed chicken fat from the top of my chilled stock. I turn on some music, maybe Blue Rodeo's "Lost Together" or Jim Cuddy's "Pull Me Through." Hello, Jim, I always say as his voice fills my house and I begin to chop again, the same ingredients I used for the broth yesterday—onions, celery, carrots, and garlic. This time, I chop them into nice soup-size pieces because they will become part of the finished product, not the garbage. Then I sauté the chopped veggies in olive or canola oil. The taste of olive oil is best, but canola has a higher smoke point. Butter works too. When the onions are soft and translucent, but not brown, I add enough fresh stock to fill the pot almost to the top. The remainder goes into the freezer for when I want to make soup in less than two days.

When the contents in my pot reach a gentle boil, I add a handful of orzo. Orzo is a great little pasta because it swells nicely, but doesn't get mushy like other noodles. Then I chop up some of the tender chicken meat and add it to the pot. I return the rest of the chicken to the refrigerator, hoping that the other person who lives in my house will make his meals out of it for a few days. I season the soup and let it simmer until lunchtime. At noon, I set a place for one and serve myself a generous portion. I raise a big spoonful to my mouth and give it a little blow before it goes in. Cornucopia soup. Cor-new-coh-pee-ah.

Survival Gear

When my feet start to hurt inside my shoes, I know why. My big toes have a strong tendency to become ingrown. The nails dig into the skin around them, creating wounds my body inflicts upon itself. I ignore the pain at first, but if I let it go for too long, what comes next will be agony. Sometimes I resort to holding my face in my hands. I bury my cheeks into my palms, let my index and middle fingers rise up to cradle my eyeballs. I massage the bones of my eye sockets, hoping my consciousness will go someplace else. But it usually goes right back to my big toes. So I fish around in my nail kit for my scissors, and start the rude surgery to extract the miscreant chunks of keratin.

My scissors are good ones, matte stainless steel, made in Italy, ever so slightly curved at the pointed end. I've had them for only a few years. My previous pair was confiscated at airport security when I forgot to take them out of my carry-on bag. I bought a new pair as soon as I returned home. In my survival kit, nail scissors are an essential tool.

I sometimes think of what I carry around with me and what I put on my body each day as my survival kit. The costumes we

clothe ourselves in show the personae we present to our world—
at least we hope they do. The things we put in our pockets and
our bags are what we need to survive as that costumed being.

With my home surgery complete, relief is instantaneous.
I always take a moment to observe the offending piece of nail—
its curve reminds me of a bow missing its string and arrow.
Sometimes a small remnant of bronze nail polish still adheres
to the flatter straight section. I'll hold the fragment up to the
light and examine its wounding edge. At the unpolished end,
the inner curve so recently embedded in my toe is sharp, like the
blade of an X-Acto knife.

My feet have both taken me into danger and saved me from
it. It was around Halloween about four decades ago that I had
my first near-death experience, or at least my first awareness of
having a close call with potential violence. When I was a foolish
young woman of twenty-one, I was walking alone one night in
a dimly lit suburb of London, England. I'd been shopping on
Carnaby Street and was all dressed up in a new costume.

I didn't think of it as a costume at the time. I thought
of it as the best outfit I'd ever had: a pair of purple plus-four
pants—also known as knickerbockers back then—complete with
purple stockings, a long tunic-style purple pullover sweater—
also known as a jumper in Great Britain—and a purple felt hat,
gaucho-cowboy style. On my feet I wore new black platform
shoes with big shiny silver buckles. At my waist, I cinched in
my long sweater with a wide black belt. Over my purple get-up,
I wore a leopard-print coat. My hair was long and blonde at the
time. I walked tall under my gaucho hat that night, feeling like a
Canadian version of Marianne Faithfull.

But I was lost. I'd taken the last train from the centre of
London. As it neared the end of the line, I grew nervous because
I realized that I wasn't exactly sure where I was going. I con-
sulted the small map I had in my pocket, and the piece of paper

on which my friend Jean's cousin had written directions to her house. I got off the train, picked a direction, and started walking. The further I got from the train station, the darker the night became. A small car pulled up beside me. The man inside asked me where I was going. I told him the address. He said he could take me there. I hesitated, but he opened the door and patted the seat beside him, so I got in the car.

Within seconds of closing the door, I knew I'd made a mistake. As he shifted the car into gear, he leaned over and smiled in my face. He smelled of stale beer. I felt itchy all over my body.

"I've changed my mind," I said. "Let me out."

"Not to worry, luv," he said. "I'll look after you."

He leaned his smiling face in close to mine again. His teeth were crooked and stained.

I started screaming. I flailed at the windshield with my new black patent purse and kicked at the dashboard with my platform shoes. After only a minute or so of this hullabaloo, the driver pulled over and pushed me out of his car. "You're too much trouble," I heard him say as he squealed off down the road. An hour later, I found Jean's cousin's house.

I've never told anyone this story before. I remember waking up the next morning feeling like an idiot. For the first time in my life, I realized that a hard truth was my reality. Women did not have the same freedom as men in this world. We always have to be looking over our shoulders. Maybe that man wasn't dangerous. I'll never know for certain. But my bones tell me that I had a close call. I decided at the time that I could never tell anyone about this experience, especially not my mother. She would have been furious at me for being so stupid.

There's an old black-and-white picture of me with my father. I'm little, probably not yet two years old. In the background, I can see a radiator, heavy flowered curtains, and a window showing leafless trees against the sky. I'm in the foreground, wearing a pristine white dress and a small white ribbon in my hair. I'm between my father's knees with my back towards the camera, but I've turned around to look at the photographer, who has probably called out my name. I'm not quite smiling, but I'm not frowning either. My eyes are wide and round. I look curious, as if I'm taking the opportunity to study the photographer or the camera from the safe haven of my father's nearness.

Dad is sitting in a chair, wearing a light-coloured suit, a white shirt, and a dark tie. He's bending over me and seems to be whispering in my ear. His right hand is around my waist. His left hand holds a drink, a short tumbler containing ice and a liquid. His hair is thick and looks darker than it really was. It's parted on the left, along the scalp scar from when he cracked his head open at a swimming pool, diving off a high board and landing on a low one. His eyes aren't visible in this picture, but the viewer can see that he was a handsome young man in his mid-twenties. He's probably saying something to me. When I look at this picture, I can almost hear his voice saying my name, the way he used to say it when I was small: "Myrlie." He's the only person who ever called me that. No one else would dare.

The details of the photo tell me that we must be visiting my grandparents, maybe for Sunday night dinner. I'm almost certain it's my grandparents' house because my mother would never have picked those curtains, and my father is dressed up. As a salesman, his job was to impress people he met so they would want to do business with him. Thus my father's workday wear was a suit, a white shirt, and a tie. Every weekday that's what he put on when he got up in the morning. Outside of work, he only wore a suit to funerals and weddings—or to visit his parents.

In another black-and-white photo of the same vintage, I see similar curtains and some tall potted plants in the background. I look like I'm the same age I was in the other picture, but I'm wearing a different dress, probably one my grandparents bought for me. My mother always made certain that her children wore the clothes her in-laws gave us when we visited. But there is no sibling "us" yet. I'm still the only child of my parents. I see my knobby little knees far below the hem of my dress, which is almost too small for me. I must be growing fast. I'm standing between my mother and my grandmother, who are both seated. Mom is wearing a full-skirted dress in a floral print. Granny is all white: her hair is white, her teeth are white, her dress is white. She smiles at the camera and holds one of my small hands in both of hers. Mom is also smiling as she looks down at me. Her lustrous dark hair is long and shiny. Her fingernails are painted a dark colour. I can see her wedding ring—a main staple of her survival kit. Her eyes aren't visible, but viewers of this photo can see that she is beautiful. I am not smiling. I am a serious-looking child. My eyes are wide and round as I gaze directly into the camera.

I've looked at this picture countless times over the years. Only recently did I notice the cuffed trousers of a man's pant leg in the lower right corner. The trousers are neatly pressed. From the angle of the leg, the man would be sitting with his legs crossed. Not many men sit like that, but my grandfather sometimes did. Which means the photographer was probably my father, calling my name. I wonder what the camera that made these images possible looked like.

I once bought a ravishing witch cape made out of shiny black satin and featuring a wonderful red stand-up collar. Thinking about it now, I realize it must have been a vampire cape, but on the day I bought it, I thought it was a witch cape. I found a marvellous tall pointy hat with a great wide brim to go with it. My intention was to wear this glorious get-up to a surprise party for my brother-in-law, whose birthday is on Halloween. We had a three-hour drive from Edmonton to their home and arrived mid-afternoon. When I went to get dressed for the party, I discovered that I'd forgotten to pack my costume. In fact, I'd forgotten to pack my husband's costume as well. My sister is a resourceful person. She lent me a spare witch costume she had on hand, and my husband wore my brother-in-law's red bath-robe along with a devil mask to the party.

I never did wear my exquisite witch costume. After storing it in my closet for a decade or so, I gave it away. I feel stiff in costumes, like I'm in a body that doesn't know what to do with what's been put on it. Creating unique Halloween costumes is a challenge for me, an always excruciating exercise. Coming up with someone I'd like to impersonate for this one evening of the year is always a dilemma that brings nothing but a blank into my head. I have no problem dressing myself up as me, but dressing myself as someone else is a conundrum, as if putting my body into alien clothing will leave me with no idea of how to behave.

Halloween hasn't always been like that for me. As a kid, I was eager to dress up. With my face painted and wearing a costume my mother created under a warm winter jacket, I carried a white pillowcase in my hand as I went out the door with my siblings on the last night of October every year. Our parents didn't go with us. They stayed home, where Dad watched television and Mom handed out candy. We'd walk as many streets of our neighbourhood as we could, venturing up to familiar and unfamiliar doorsteps, calling out "Halloween Apples!" We didn't like saying "Trick or Treat." We wanted treats. Why issue an invitation for someone to trick us instead? When we got tired or our pillowcases got too heavy, we'd drag them back home again.

After we'd shed our witch or hobo or pirate costumes, and handed our orange UNICEF boxes over to Mom, we'd spread our loot out on the living-room floor to see who got the most. We didn't like getting apples, and usually threw out any that turned up in our bags. Not because of razor-blade scares—our mother said that would never happen in our neighbourhood—but because the ones we got were usually bruised with brown spots, and some were mushy. Mom allowed us to eat a few pieces of candy before we went to bed on Halloween night. The rest of our loot went back into our pillowcases, which we'd store in our bedroom closets until either the candy ran out, or Mom got rid of it so she could have the pillowcases back.

In Mexico and other Spanish-speaking countries, November the second is *El Día de los Muertos*, Day of the Dead, a fun celebration of death. Smiling skulls show up everywhere. In preparation, people clean up the area around their loved ones' graves and decorate them with bright yellow marigolds, maybe some fruit and toys for the children. On the day, families and friends gather at the cemetery, bringing food and drink and flowers with them for a graveside picnic. They believe the deceased are there with them, laughing and partying, their souls as present as their bones.

I don't remember ever dressing up as a skeleton on Halloween, but I should have. I like the bones of the body. My dad and I used to sing a little song around the house, impromptu bursts that could have happened any time of the year, but probably a lot around Halloween. Dad would usually start this singing ritual, maybe on a Saturday morning as he refilled his coffee cup from the percolator on the counter. We liked the words, the song's simple beat, the rhythmic sensation as the lyrics travelled up and down the body, up and down "dem bones, dem bones, dem dry bones."

The "Dry Bones" song is an old spiritual, but we seldom bothered with the "Hear the Word of the Lord" refrain. We'd begin by following the song's lyrics as written and listening carefully as we sang. We liked to catch each other messing up on the order of the bones. Dad might sing "the foot bone's connected to the heel bone, the heel bone's connected to the leg bone..." and I'd say "You missed the ankle bone!" Sometimes we reconstructed that melodic skeleton and our neck bones ended up connected to our hip bones, our thigh bones connected to our shoulder bones, or our head bones connected to nothing at all. Sometimes we brought in bones ignored by the lyrics as sung by the Delta Rhythm Boys or the Lennon Sisters. How about a belly button bone connected to an ear lobe bone? Or a chin bone connected to the butt bone?

Music was the great reliever in the house I grew up in. Singing along with the music coming out of the old hi-fi in the living room felt good, whether we belted out the words or quietly mouthed them. Singing was a big exhalation, a release in a household where unshared emotions always lurked just below the surface, liable to erupt at any moment. Like many of their generation, my parents' expectation was that we would keep any unruly feelings under control. Moody or pouty behaviour on our part evoked a "who do you think you are, the Queen of Sheba?" parental response. In those instances, the best strategy was a quick retreat to a parent-free part of the house.

Halloween, once known as All Hallows Eve, is a hand-me-down occasion, derived from All Souls' Day, which came from pagan festivals similar to *El Día de los Muertos*, but without the picnics and the laughter. Throughout the centuries, the Roman Empire and Celtic folklore contributed some lighter elements to the occasion, such as costumes and bonfires and pranks.

Like Easter without the big Christian narrative, Halloween is a transition time. Centuries ago, people believed it was a time when the newly deceased darted around in the air, caught in that dangerous moment after death when souls are unsettled about where to go next. In what may be the first Halloween costumes, people disguised themselves in case those flighty souls were also disgruntled souls seeking vengeance against those who had disgruntled them. Costumes were their survival gear.

I wasn't very good at creating costumes for my children when they were small. One year I cut face holes in three white sheets and tied one of their father's ties loosely around each of their necks. The picture I still have of their eyes showing wide in the slashed holes tells me that all three were smiling under their sheets. Lucky me. My lovely trio smiled a lot. Yet whenever I look at that photo, I'm appalled at myself. Really? Sheets? And those neckties? They could have strangled themselves.

After they grew up and no longer needed me to create ghost costumes out of old sheets, my Halloween became very simple. For many years, I still carved a pumpkin, just for old times' sake. I tried to give him—yes, my pumpkins were always male—a different look each year. Sometimes I carved his mouth into a manic smile, sometimes a scowl. Once I left one eye shut, hoping that he'd look like he was winking. Instead, he looked like a one-eyed pumpkin that I'd forgotten to finish carving. A few years ago, I decided to forgo pumpkins forever and bought a plastic skull with a light inside it. At about five o'clock on Halloween afternoon, I pull it out of the crawl space, dust it off, plunk it down on the table in the front window, and plug it in.

Then I get the Halloween candy I still buy every year, and put it in a bowl by the front door. When I go shopping for that candy, I tell myself to buy the kind that neither my husband nor I like, the sticky lollipops and that hard toffee stuff. And every year, I come home with the kind we do like, the Kit Kat bars and mini boxes of Smarties. I always buy enough to hand out to about a hundred kids. And we always get about ten, so my husband and I spend the month of November eating our leftover candy. It's a ritual that needs changing. One of these years, we're going to follow through on our next plan. Buy no candy, turn out the lights, and don't answer the door. I can do it. If I put my mind to it.

I nearly drowned in France once. On the Ardèche River. My husband and I were travelling with friends who decided that we should take a paddling trip, they in kayaks, my husband and I in their canoe. They were very experienced river people. We were not.

The first part of the trip was tranquil. Then we got into some rapids. Our friends had told us to expect this and how to handle it. We negotiated the first few patches well. Then we came to stronger rapids, and the next thing I knew I was in the water. I didn't panic because our friends had said that this might happen, and had told us what to do if it did. We laughed as we surfaced and draped ourselves over the bottom of our canoe. The rapids had spilled us out into a calm part of the river, so it wasn't too long before we'd fetched our paddles, righted the canoe, and carried on, wet but happy, almost relieved that we'd had a dumping experience and would go home with a story to tell. As we paddled along the next stretch of river, our friends offered more advice. If it happened again, we were to hold tight onto our paddles.

We rounded a bend and went headlong into another stretch of rapids, these ones more menacing, their white foam spraying high and wide. Sitting in the front of the canoe, I saw nothing but swirling water. The rapids spun our canoe into a small cove bounded by a rock wall. We flipped. As I went under, I kept a firm grip on my paddle with one hand. Right away, I could feel that these rapids were very different from the first ones. Instead of spitting us out into calmer waters, they trapped us in their swirl, pulling us around and around, flinging us within arm's reach of the steep slippery rock wall. My husband, with his stronger muscle mass, hauled himself out into the main river and up onto flat rocks on the other side where our friends were. I was still stuck in the swirl. With one hand engaged in a death grip on my paddle, I couldn't free myself from the pull of the rapids. The current kept sucking me under.

When I went under for the third time, it occurred to me that I might never see my children again, that it was so stupid of me to leave them like this. The next time I surfaced, I heard my husband's voice: "Let go of the goddamned paddle!" As soon as I did that, and had two arms to work with, I managed to propel myself to calmer water. Soon I stood shivering beside my husband on the rocks, going into mild shock. My friend took off her wetsuit and stuffed my body into it. That was a costume I was happy to wear for a while.

We survived our trip down the Ardèche River. But I cannot escape the story. We see those friends seldom now, not because of the river, but because of distance and changing lives. When we do get together, our Ardèche adventure always comes up in conversation. Hearing the story makes me uncomfortable, and I once asked them all not to tell it any more. But here I am telling it myself. I survived to tell it because of the words I heard in that moment, the same words I use now to build my narrative of that day.

Words and pictures—survival gear for our stories.

Wearing Black

Several years ago I went to a funeral for a woman I'd never met. I went because her daughter is my friend. In the middle of an afternoon, in the middle of a pew, in the middle of a chapel filling up with people, I waited for the service to begin. I wore my good black suit and my red velvet scarf. I wore the scarf because black at a cocktail party is sophisticated, but black on its own at a funeral is too bleak.

The usual questions didn't take long to come into my head. *Why do we go to funerals? What are funerals for?* I know the practical reasons. Funeral traditions are the methods we use to dispose of bodies and comfort families. We go to funerals because we are still alive, and someone else is not. We go for the living, not the dead. We go because we are expected to go. "Make it stop," a friend said recently after an intense series of funerals. But funerals never stop. They keep coming. And we keep going.

While waiting for the service to begin, I looked down at the program I'd received at the door. The cover featured a photograph of the deceased. I saw my friend's face in her mother's portrait. We had occasionally talked about our mothers, especially our relationships with them, but I'd never imagined what my friend's mother looked like. I saw that she had been a beautiful woman.

During the funeral, her husband, children, and grandchildren took turns speaking about how she influenced their lives. One said that she used to be a gifted pianist. That's when I noticed a piano stool sitting beside the pulpit, a sheet of music on a stand beside it. My eyes kept falling on those items, moving from the piano stool to the sheet of music, and back to the stool again. Through them and the words her family spoke that day, a dead woman I'd never known came alive for me.

My mother was also a pianist and, in her later years, she played the organ. She'd been a young mom. I was born two weeks before her twentieth birthday. As I grew up, ours was a push-pull relationship, one pushing away as the other pulled in. Sometimes I did the pushing, sometimes she did. When I was a little girl, I adored my father: Mom made me do chores, but Dad made me laugh. Even before dementia ate away the last four years of her life, I think I knew that she and I would part uneasily.

I once asked Mom what I was like as a child. She looked at me for a long moment before answering. "Wilful," she said. "You were very wilful." In my adult years, during casual conversations with friends, I sometimes said that I didn't much like my mother, but I never felt comfortable when I said it: as if I were betraying myself somehow.

My mother's death wasn't a surprise, but it was a shock. We knew it was coming, just not so soon. I thought I was ready for the day the inevitable would happen. I was wrong about that. Mom left no instructions about what we should do after she died, other than a yellow scrap of paper on which she'd scribbled the words "no funeral." I was skeptical. What my mother said and what she meant were often quite different. Sometimes when she said "Fine with me," her jaw would be tight, and I'd suspect that whatever it was wasn't fine with her at all. If we didn't have a funeral, or at least some kind of service, I feared she might float around our lives, clenching her teeth and haunting us forever.

My sister and I talked on the phone about what to do. "Why don't we wait a few months before doing anything?" I suggested. She said she'd talk to the others. The next day, she called back. Some of the family wanted a funeral, and they wanted it sooner rather than later. We settled on the following Friday for the service. As a family, we were no longer religious. We also knew that my mother, a longtime Anglican, had turned away from organized religion in the last decades of her life. So we decided on a short simple event, a memorial gathering, informal and secular.

We divided up the immediate tasks. My sister would organize the cremation and funeral home arrangements. I was to write the obituary and come up with an outline for the service. At first, I thought my assigned chores were straightforward jobs. I was wrong about that, too. Without the model of a church service to follow, or the presence of a solemn minister to tell me what to do, I felt adrift, out on a choppy lake with no motor, no paddle, no sail.

The first funeral I remember is one I did not attend. After my maternal grandfather died, I expected to go to his service. My mother shook her head. My uncle had decided that funerals were no place for children. I was indignant. I wasn't a child. I was almost fifteen.

The first funeral I did attend was for my great-aunt, who died a few years after my grandfather. By then I was all grown-up—going on seventeen. The details of that service are lost to me now, but I do remember the cemetery afterwards. I walked over to the marker indicating my grandfather's grave, perhaps feeling cold and shivery, perhaps thinking about what it might be like to lie underground, perhaps imagining worms crawling in the bony sockets that used to house his eyeballs.

In the next few decades, most of the funerals I went to were for aunts and uncles, the older generation of my family. Depending on how close I was to the deceased, the experience of being a mourner stayed with me for days, or weeks, or in the case of my father's funeral, the rest of my life.

With only five days until my mother's service, I sat at my computer in my small home office. My sister called to say that the funeral home needed the obituary right away. I promised to have it ready later that afternoon.

Flipping through the morning newspaper, I studied all the funeral listings and jotted down the most repeated words and phrases: "beloved," "cherished," "forever in our hearts." Good words, expected words, words that are either too much or not enough. With my list beside me, my fingers sat poised on my keyboard. But they wouldn't move. So I picked up a notebook, grabbed a pen, and dove into my favourite living-room chair. Throwing a blanket over my legs, I settled in and finally began to write. "With great sadness, the family announces the passing of..."

I once went to a funeral for someone I didn't know well. I went because, through family connections, I was expected to be there. Mourners mingled in the foyer of the chapel before the service. I stood off to the side, watching them exchange sad smiles and embraces. I decided that people hug differently at funerals than they do on other occasions. They tilt their heads as they walk towards each other, fall into a slow squeeze, and hold it a little longer than normal. Women continue the hug even when it's over, holding each other's hands for a few more seconds. Men embrace briefly, then clap each other on the back and shoulder as they step away.

The deceased had a large family. I didn't know any of them well, some of them not at all. I listened to his children talk about the father they'd lost. I didn't recognize him. To me, he had been someone of little presence and few words, someone who sat in a corner, disappeared into the recesses of crowded rooms. The man they described told stories at the dinner table, took his children and grandchildren fishing, played the guitar, and sang to them at bedtime. I could not find him in my memory of the person I'd known: I wished I'd met the other guy.

After I finished writing Mom's obituary, I e-mailed it to my siblings for their approval. Waiting to hear back from them, I sat in my living room staring out the window. It was more than a week into April, and snow still covered our front yard, but the maple tree had buds on its branches. I sat there long enough for daylight to fade, acutely aware of my new situation as the oldest living person in the family my parents created. My parents had not been together for a long time, and I wondered if they were now. I counted the years and realized that twenty-five had passed since my father's death. Remembering that his funeral service did not include a eulogy, I returned to my computer to do a search for the year of my mother's birth.

My mother was born two and a half months before the stock market crash that began the Great Depression. Hit songs of the year were "Singin' in the Rain" and "Makin' Whoopee." 1929 was the last year of the Roaring Twenties, and the first year of the Academy Awards. When I was a child, my mother and I always watched the Oscars together. She loved every minute of that endless show, which was strange because she rarely went to the movies.

*My mother was born in the same year as Jacqueline Lee
Bouvier. Thirty-four years later, I sat beside Mom, transfixed
in front of the television, as we watched the surreal events
following President Kennedy's assassination. I felt as if we
didn't move from the couch for days. When the camera showed
Jackie Kennedy standing on the White House steps in her trim
black coat and flowing veil, holding hands with her two young
children, I heard my mother say, "She and I are exactly the
same age."*

The most elegant funeral I ever attended took place in a cath-
edral with a soaring ceiling, stained-glass windows, three aisles,
and a choir loft. The deceased was too young—just into his
fifties—so the church overflowed with mourners. An organist
played as we assembled. A robed attendant entered from a side
door and lit the tapered candles that stood sentinel beside the
raised altar. Hushed chatter rose to a steady hum as we waited
for the service to begin. Then the hum faded to silence.

I will never forget his family's calm faces as they followed
the casket down the centre aisle. The control they had over
their emotions was almost too difficult to watch. The service
included prayers and several eulogies. People laughed and
cried. The choir sang "I Know That My Redeemer Liveth" and
"Amazing Grace."

Afterwards, the congregation emptied out of the church
and lingered on the steps under bright August sunshine. At
the reception, I watched his wife smile and talk to everyone
in the crowded room. I thought how exhausted she must be,
but I too had to speak to her, just for a moment. Her serenity
was magnetic.

I soon discovered that writing a eulogy takes a lot of time.
First you have to travel back. Then you have to write what you

discovered on that journey of the mind. I gathered the facts of my mother's life, but the words would not flow. My brain groped for images of how her years had evolved. I sent off an e-mail asking my siblings for pictures. Then I went downstairs to the crawl space under my living room and dragged out a large bin of photographs, hitting my head on a joist as I backed out.

For hours, I rummaged through images I hadn't looked at in years, many of them old black-and-white photos in which my mother's glorious dark hair glowed and her cheekbones soared. In many close-ups, I saw her luminous pearl necklace, the one my paternal grandparents gave her after baby number two. Or was it number three? In one picture, I recognized the front steps of her family's summer cabin. Mom looks to be about fifteen and has one arm draped around a large shaggy sheepdog. His tongue lolls out of his mouth and he looks like he's smiling. I remembered my mother talking about how much she loved that dog. *What was his name? Buddy? Butch?*

I found a faded colour picture of our whole family, my youngest sister held high in my father's arms, my other three siblings clustered around my mother. I stand on the right edge of the group, beside Dad. I noticed that I'd placed myself as far away as I could from Mom. We must have had an argument that day.

As I settled back in front of my computer, I wondered how old my mother was when she went to her first funeral, and whose it was. Maybe it was for her own mother, who died unexpectedly when Mom was only seventeen, rendering her the youngest child of a grieving widower.

> *My grandfather was a successful businessman who owned an auto dealership. My mother used to tell me that she always had her own car and a fur coat as a teenager. Mom was nineteen years old when she married Dad. Over the next fourteen years,*

they had five children. The house we lived in was built for a much smaller family, and often felt as if its walls bulged outwards. I'd like to say it was always a happy place, but I can't. Sometimes my father wasn't home enough. Sometimes my mother was testy. Sometimes she was sad. But when she was at peace with her world, that house was as cheery as a brass band marching on a clear day, trombones and French horns glinting in the sun.

Several years ago, an old friend from my high-school days fell sick. His illness progressed fast, and his death was a harsh blow for those close to him. I hadn't seen him for years. During the funeral, I listened as his daughter, mother of his first grandchild, still an infant, talked about how angry she was. She read a letter she'd written to her father as she sat beside his deathbed. How could he leave her? How could he go without watching his grandson learn to walk and talk and skip rocks across a lake?

My friend's family ended that service with a slide show of photographs. I watched the pictures glide by, welcoming the sight of that familiar face, that trouble-seeking grin. Then he aged. I was surprised to see he'd become completely white-haired in his fifties. Later I wondered why I was surprised. Had I looked in a mirror lately?

His daughter's words stayed with me for days afterwards. I kept thinking about how she gave voice to her anger, an emotion not normally expressed at funerals. Her father was a man with flaws, like all of us. Instead of idealizing him in her eulogy, she talked to the man her father had been as if he were sitting in the front row, listening to every word.

Three days before my mother's service, the carpet covering the floor of my home office was no longer visible, hidden under piles of pictures and photograph albums. I was now in mother overload. I couldn't walk from my bedroom to the kitchen without seeing her face. But what face? The younger stern one or the older furrowed one? They blurred together. I made cup after cup of herbal tea to take back to my desk, where I sat listening to the silence around me.

The house I grew up in was rarely silent. Sounds and smells filled almost every waking hour. Oatmeal simmering in a pot. Bacon sizzling in the electric frying pan. The television in the front room. The radio in the kitchen. Children shouting. At each other. At her. "Mom, I'm leaving." "Mom, I'm home." "Mom, when's supper ready?" "Mom, we're out of shampoo."

On weekend mornings, the clamour changed, softened, as we listened for my father's deep singing voice. He sounded like Louis Armstrong, but he could croon like Perry Como too. When he sang, my mother usually smiled.

As the oldest, I was my mother's helper. She taught me to do what she did. Sweep the kitchen floor. Dust the furniture. Iron the tea towels and my father's boxer shorts. His business shirts were too difficult for me to manage, so she did those herself.

One day, I was at the ironing board when Dad came home from work. He asked if I knew what Mom wanted for her upcoming birthday. I was grumpy. "I don't know," I said, "but we sure could use a new iron."

When the day came, she opened her present and let out a deep sigh. I felt terrible. I didn't think my father would actually buy her an iron for her birthday. We shared a sheepish look. After that, my mother never received another domestic appliance as a gift from Dad. And she never got one from me, either.

I didn't wear black to my father's funeral those many years ago. To this day, I can still see my outfit. A yellow blazer and an orange plaid skirt. My father didn't like his daughters to wear black, and that yellow blazer was my favourite piece of clothing.

The July day was a Calgary scorcher. My head hurt. I still didn't believe it. My father was dead. He was only sixty. How could he be dead? Yes, he drank too much alcohol and smoked too many cigarettes. And yes, he hadn't looked well this past year. But he and my mother had separated only six months earlier, so I didn't expect him to look good. I had expected him to get better once he adjusted to his new life as a single man.

The funeral happened fast, only four days after they found him on the floor of his apartment. The church was full. The service was short. The minister talked about not questioning the life lived, but celebrating the universal gift of life itself. I don't think my father's name was mentioned.

I boarded a flight out of Calgary that night, clutching a flower I'd taken from my father's casket. The plane took off, and the tears started. Quiet tears that just wouldn't stop flowing. I didn't have a tissue. I asked the flight attendant for one. And another one. And another one. Soon she brought me a whole box. By the time my plane landed, the flower from my father's casket was petal shreds in my hands.

In the last box I dragged out of the crawl space, I found the pictures from my first wedding. I'm sandwiched between my parents. We are tanned and our faces are all teeth. I'm wearing white. My mother is in yellow. My father has a rose in his lapel. I got married in the afternoon. We had a champagne reception. By suppertime, the whole thing was over. For years afterwards, I wished we'd had a dance so that I could have danced with my new husband in front of all our guests, so that I could have danced with my father, so that everyone could have had a chance to dance at my wedding.

In the same box, I found the pictures from my second wedding. One shows me and my family all dancing in a line, kicking our feet up as if doing the can-can, our arms around each other's waists. In another shot, my parents dance together. My mother's eyes are on him. My father's eyes are on the camera, my camera.

Two days before Mom's memorial service, I began to feel acute anxiety. Weather forecasts indicated another impending April snowstorm. I was scheduled to leave the next day for the three-hour drive to Calgary, and I hadn't finished the eulogy yet. Gluing my butt to my chair, I adjusted my keyboard and sat contemplating my hands for a few moments. I spread them out in front of me, stretching each finger, making them as long as possible. My fingers are short and stubby, the knuckles wide and chunky. They are my father's hands.

My mother's hands were elegant, her fingers long and tapered, the hands of a gifted seamstress. She taught me how to sew as soon as I was big enough to sit at her black Singer sewing machine. She taught me so well that by the time I went to Home Economics classes in high school, I was making many of my own clothes. When the teacher showed us how to put in a zipper, I told her that my mother had a better way of doing it. As proof, I showed her the zipper I'd inserted the night before in the side seam of a skirt I was making for my term project. My teacher made me rip it out and do it her way.

My mother's hands had music in them. An upright piano sat in our basement next to the sewing machine. When my mother played it, she chose songs from her parents' era, songs like "Peg o' my Heart" and "My Wild Irish Rose." I don't remember ever hearing her sing along to the tunes she played.

My mother's hands also had medicine in them. They showed me how to clean the dirt out of scraped knees, how to take a toddler's temperature with the back of my wrist, how to

wrap a blanket around an injured child before rushing her to
the hospital.

My mother's hands taught me how to peel potatoes; how
to hold a baby, burp a baby, and change a diaper; how to put
pantyhose on without snagging the fabric; how to put rollers in
my hair and sleep on them overnight.

My mother taught me how to get up each morning and
take on the tasks of the day, regardless of how I'm feeling. She
gave me many skills that I've taken for granted even as I've put
them to good use in my life. I wish I'd told her that.

After I finally finished writing the eulogy, I made a slide show
of the photographs I had selected. Then I packed my funeral
clothes: my best black dress and my pearl necklace. I'd have taken
the same yellow blazer I'd worn to Dad's funeral, but it was long
gone, in one of my closet-cleaning purges.

At her death, my mother didn't have a lot of friends left,
many having died or become immobile. We didn't expect a big
crowd at her service, and we didn't get one. A few of my sister's
friends, who had known Mom for years, came. My siblings and
I were elated when her only surviving cousin walked in.

To their great credit, all my mother's grandchildren
showed up. They rearranged schedules to be there. Some flew
in from far away. Some drove on dark highways through the
mountains in an April blizzard.

At the funeral home, we mourners met in the anteroom.
A table covered with a white cloth stood inside the entrance to
the chapel. On it, we placed a portrait of my mother, her hair
perfectly styled, her smile radiant. Beside the picture, I put a tall
glass angel I'd given her a decade ago after she survived a bout
with breast cancer. Someone brought a basket for condolence
cards and a guest book. We left a space in the middle for the urn
containing her ashes.

Writing my mother's eulogy had taken me almost a whole week, but giving it took less than fifteen minutes. Saying the eulogy out loud in front of my family changed it for me. With my chosen words hanging in the air, I felt my mother as she used to be. In bidding goodbye to the difficult old woman she'd become at the end of her life, I leapt over the chasm between us. I said hello again to her younger self, jumped back in time to the days when she was the centre of my world, a centre the wilful child in me had resisted.

Then everyone had a chance to speak. When no one else rose to take the podium, I signalled for the slideshow to begin. I'd put it together backwards. Instead of starting at the beginning of her life, I started at the end. The first picture was of my elderly mother dancing at my son's wedding less than two years before her death. The last shot was a formal portrait of a solemn-faced little girl with an oversized white bow perched on the top of her head. For five minutes, we watched as my mother grew younger and younger until she disappeared into an image of her parents. We saw that she had been beautiful.

After that, we moved back into the anteroom, where a light lunch waited for us. Not until we'd eaten and were preparing to leave did we notice that my mother's urn wasn't on the table next to her portrait. The chapel attendants had forgotten to put her out. As they apologized in quiet, sincere voices, I smiled to myself. How like my mother to miss her own funeral. She hated the idea of dying.

Music on the Hill

On a January day, I stood at the top of Gallagher Park, home to Edmonton's annual folk music festival. The Park's main hill spread out below me, Cloverdale's Community League Hall looking snug under its snow-covered roof. Across the North Saskatchewan River, the city centre skyline hunkered down under leaden grey clouds that looked too heavy to stay aloft. Behind me, a bus dieselled by as it crested Connors Hill. Overhead, a helicopter buzzed past. But down on the hill, quiet prevailed. Nothing moved. The nearby ski lift was idle even though fresh snow had fallen for the past three days. On such a classic deep winter afternoon, it was difficult to picture the summer festival in action here, hard to imagine the four nights and two full days of non-stop motion and music that occupy this site just days after the August long weekend, the place where, for the past fifteen years, I've spent my annual "stay-cation," recovering from my birthday by losing myself in a hometown holiday.

The familiar phrase Edmontonians know so well, the Edmonton Folk Music Festival, is a misnomer that tends to evoke images of dishevelled singers playing battered out-of-tune guitars while singing tired versions of "Michael Row the Boat Ashore" into dated static-y microphones. This couldn't be more inaccurate. Ours is a refined festival masterpiece. It should be called the Edmonton Folk, Roots, Blues, Celtic, Bluegrass, Gospel, Pop, and World Music Festival, but the acronym EFRBCBGPWMF wouldn't have the same appealing balance as EFMF.

To us regulars, us Folkies, it's simply Folkfest. We are well aware that many other music festivals take place across the country, the continent, and the world. And we have no doubt that they are very good festivals. But we are also confident that ours rises above the rest, sets a standard to which all the others aspire. After all, every year, at least one performer stands up on a stage and says so.

For well over thirty years, Folkfest's physical home has been Edmonton's Gallagher Park. In early summer, the park spends weeks preparing for it; in late summer, it spends several more recuperating from it. The park's large hill creates a natural amphitheatre. Each summer, Folkfest's signature green-and-white striped awning rises over the Main Stage at the bottom of that ascending expanse. From there, the other stages, food concessions, beer gardens, merchandise tents, and many rows of Port-a-Potties spread east and west. During Folkfest, Gallagher Park is transformed into a city within a city, a temporary municipality governed by a dedicated team with the help of two thousand volunteers.

Folkfest has its own language, one that contains words the general public may not associate with a musical event: words like tarp and lottery and bullpen. Tarp is a key word here. Short for tarpaulin, it permeates the Folkfest air.

"Where's your tarp today?"

"How many tarps does your group have?"

"Our tarp is five down from the sound booth, right beside the cables."

Once nailed down on the hill, your tarp is your home for each day. You can walk away from it, and no one will touch anything on it. You can go for a beer or green onion cakes or CD shopping, and while you're gone, people will walk all over your tarp, but they won't help themselves to your stuff or rifle through your backpack. Maybe that's because everyone knows what's in those backpacks: blankets, sunscreen, rain gear, mosquito spray, binoculars, maybe a sandwich or two, probably a thermos of smuggled-in wine—the standard survival kit for four days of music. But maybe, just maybe, your stuff is safe on your tarp because Folkies are also on a brief respite from the outside world, a world in which an unattended backpack is an invitation to theft.

Folkfest is an oasis where more than twenty thousand people a day congregate for four consecutive days, sometimes in searing heat, sometimes in driving rain. Getting into Folkfest is an intricate multi-step endeavour. The first step is to acquire a ticket. This can be a challenge because they usually sell out the day they go on sale, sometimes in only a few hours.

The next step is a knotty one and relates to the EFMF's unique seating philosophy. Folkies bring their own seats. That's what we put on our tarps. So the seating arrangement process is in fact a tarp placement exercise. One eight-by-ten tarp accommodates eight people comfortably. That's eight people with eight low-backed chairs, eight blankets, and eight backpacks. We've had up to twelve people on our tarp. Around midnight on cool Friday or Saturday nights, the extra bodies are a comforting source of warmth.

Folkfest offers no exclusive tickets close to the performers. Those who care about where they sit in relation to the Main Stage enter a lottery to get into the tarp placement lineup.

Tickets for that lottery are not for sale. To participate in it, we lottery hopefuls have to show up each day several hours before the gates open. But we can't show up early. We have to arrive no sooner than two in the afternoon for the two-thirty draws on Thursday and Friday, and no sooner than seven in the morning for the seven-thirty draws on Saturday and Sunday. Folkfest developed this process so people wouldn't camp overnight on the streets of a residential neighbourhood, something that happened a lot in the early Folkfest years, much to the dismay of those who live in the host community of Cloverdale.

Approximately five thousand lottery tickets are available each day. Have you ever been one of five thousand people attempting to arrive at one spot in a residential area all at the same time? It's something to see. People lurk a few blocks away, in back alleys, between parked cars, or behind hedges and trees. As the appointed time nears, we lurkers stream in from all directions. Soon a volunteer wielding a megaphone directs us to converge on an opening in an orange snow fence. As we funnel in, another volunteer hands us a coloured paper tag with the name of a festival performer printed on it. Then we spill into the lottery holding area, known to all as the bullpen. And the trading begins.

Tag trading is a key step in a successful lottery strategy. Our regular group consists of eight people. That gives us eight paper tags, which we pool together. If we have two tags bearing the same performer's name, we start trading with other bullpenners until we have eight different names. Then we wait until the volunteer with the megaphone starts the draw.

The bullpen is an active place. While waiting, people chat, drink coffee, and get their tarps ready. They take them out of their backpacks, shake them out, and repack them. Many discussions ensue, often concerning the most efficient way to carry a tarp for a quick lay-down.

"Fold it lengthwise. Tuck it under your arm."

"Roll it up. Then just fling it out."

"We need a spring-loaded tarp that flips out flat in a split second."

The volunteer with the megaphone starts the draw by calling out the first name. For example, she'll say "Rodney Crowell!" and a small cheer will go up from the thirty or forty or fifty people who have Rodney Crowell tags. Everyone else groans. The winners file out of the bullpen, where more Folkfest volunteers organize them into the lineup that will eventually go through the main gate. The volunteer with the megaphone keeps calling out names until no one is left in the bullpen.

The lottery process is both flawed and fun. One of the most fun things about it is standing in the bullpen talking about how flawed it is.

"They should do it online."

"They should grid the hill into eight-by-ten sections. Like a football field. Give each tarp spot a number. Do an electronic draw and just e-mail everyone their tarp location."

"They probably haven't thought of that. We should write a letter."

"We should. We will."

We never do.

As the days and nights of the festival progress, the bullpen mood changes. Thursday and Friday bullpens are filled with bright-eyed alert Folkies. But performances on the Main Stage go on until well after midnight on Friday and Saturday nights. This means that the Saturday and Sunday seven o'clock bullpens are full of half-awake, unshowered Folkies clutching at coffee cups, some with shaky hands. Those coffee cups might come from Tim Hortons or Starbucks or the bearers' own cupboards. Folkies are a socially diverse demographic.

When the draw is complete, only one person from each tarp waits in the lottery lineup. This person is the tarp placer.

Everyone else goes home until the music starts. Being the tarp placer is a memorable experience. Once the lottery is over, a sense of calm comes over the lineup. We pull out our chairs and sit down. We chat to our neighbours about what performers we want to see, or which food concession has the best lentil curry or naan bread or butter chicken. Volunteers come along to take our tickets and turn them into colourful wristbands. Other volunteers sell programs. We buy them and plan our festival days, consulting with each other. About ten minutes before the gates open, new volunteers get us out of our chairs and ready to go. And then comes the sound we've been waiting for—the squeal of bagpipes. The gates are open.

In the early years of Folkfest, this moment was called "running the tarp." People burst through the gates from both the top and bottom of the hill, sprinting to get to the area in front of the Main Stage ahead of the crowd. Back in those days, some older Folkies hired young fast legs to do the crucial dash for them. Running the tarp was eventually banned after the injuries that were bound to happen happened.

These days, tarps must be walked in. We form an orderly herd. Volunteers surround the herd, monitoring it to make sure no one's walk accidently turns into a run, which would then trigger a stampede. We walk as fast as we can while wearing backpacks and carrying chairs. As we get closer to our destination, we know that even the volunteer brigade won't be able to stop the run that breaks out during the last rush.

If I'm the tarp placer when we've been drawn in the fourth or fifth lottery group, I'm relaxed. Our tarp will be a ways up the hill, so the pressure is off. But if I'm the tarp placer in the coveted first group, that's not the case. The closer to the Main Stage, the more intense the competition for each square inch is. I know it's going to be a crush when we get onto the hill. I know it's all about timing. Everything has to happen fast. I'm excited and nervous. I don't chat with my lineup neighbours. I fidget with the tarp. I fold it and unfold it. I practice holding it under one arm, my backpack on my back, my chair in my other hand. I hydrate myself. I make sure my shoelaces are tied tight. I take many deep breaths.

The walk takes three or four minutes. To keep up with the group, I have to walk fast because I have short legs. When I see the dance area fence come into view, I veer wide because I don't want to get blocked on the inside. Once clear of the fence, I sprint to a patch of unclaimed grass. I don't look around because there's no time for second-guessing. I drop my chair and throw down the tarp. I spread it out fast and guard my corners so no one overlaps them. Only when I'm satisfied that I've claimed our full eight-by-ten territory do I look to see where we are. Only then do I hammer tent nails through the tarp's grommets into the grass. At this point, volunteers might come along with tape measures to ensure that oversized tarps aren't taking up more than the allotted eight-by-ten space. This is the only time I've ever heard cross words at Folkfest.

Then all is calm. The main crowds haven't yet arrived, and the music won't start for a while. Only the tarp placers, volunteers, and stage crews are here. For the next hour, the site is as quiet as it will ever be. On a Thursday or Friday afternoon, I'll stroll through the food concession area and plan my dinner options. On a Saturday or Sunday morning, I'll get a latte, sit in the sun, and reach for my program. Before long, I'll make my first performance selection and walk my chair over to its designated side stage. This gets me a front row seat. I've earned it. I'm the tarp placer. And I know that when I meet up with my tarp mates later, they will all thank me for our spot. It's a rule on our tarp. Complaints about where the tarp is located are not allowed. No matter where it is, everyone thanks the tarp placer, because we all know what it took to get it there.

Four days at Folkfest always result in four different tarp spots. We've been close, and we've been far away. The benefit of being closer to the Main Stage is obvious: the artists and their activities fill our visual frame. Everything happening on the hill behind us fades into the background. The benefit of being further back is that the whole scene becomes the experience: the Main Stage, the constant movement of people, the backdrop of downtown Edmonton as it changes in the light of the setting sun, as the moon rises, as the stars come out above us.

One year and four months after my mother's death, as Folkfest weekend approached, I was tired and distracted. After the funeral, we had moved my mother's ashes to my sister's house. And there they stayed, stored in a closet, with no consensus among her offspring on what to do with her remains. With both our parents gone, my siblings and I had little to say to each other. I've since discovered that this is not unusual when the second parent goes. But it was unusual for me. I felt like I'd lost not only my mother, but my entire birth family as well. The family we used to be no longer existed.

From the outside, my life probably looked fine. On the inside, it was erratic. Some days, I wafted through a mountain of emotions, never settling long on any particular one. Other days, I was empty. As the oldest in my family, I was keenly aware of my place in the continuum of life, of my position far closer to the death end than the birth end. My head played out unfinished conversations with my mother that would be forever on hold. I talked to her often, going over what I should have said, what I wanted to hear her say in return. But all I heard was silence.

And my inner music stopped. All my life, both my body and mind have responded to music in typically human ways— tapping toes, drumming fingers, a nodding head, swaying hips, thoughts lost in beats and lyrics. In my daily routines, I surrounded myself with music, turned it on whenever I was at home, hummed as I walked, fell asleep to it at night. Since my mother's death, all that changed. My toes were still, my hips stiff. I worked through my days in a quiet house, fell asleep only to the sounds of my rambling thoughts, and woke up to the same thoughts several times a night. When I did hear music in the background of my life, it hurt my ears, like an alien language I no longer wanted to understand. I simply didn't *feel* music anymore.

So I stood in the first Folkfest bullpen of the year daunted by the prospect of the next four days, by the whole overwhelming process, by the ebullience of life ahead, by the wealth of music I knew I would hear. In fact, I wasn't sure I could listen to any music at all. I felt my breath getting shorter as the trading of lottery tags went on around me.

The day was sunny. People chatted and laughed. I saw my friend's mouths moving, but I couldn't hear their words. Mosquitoes buzzed at my ears. It happened fast. One minute I was standing still. The next minute, I bolted, telling the puzzled volunteers guarding the bullpen's entrance that they had to let me out because I was sick. And I was. I felt nauseous and dizzy as I ran for the sanctuary of my car, where I sat in the quiet until I stopped hyperventilating. I drove home, almost going through a red light on the way. In my bedroom, I lay down with my shoes still on and put a cold cloth on my forehead.

That evening, I did return to the hill for the Thursday performances. On the tarp, I sat quietly with my friends as the performers took to the Main Stage. I remember feeling detached from the whole thing, although I did take notice when Alberta's Corb Lund took to the stage. It's difficult not to enjoy a personable young man entertaining a hill full of eager music aficionados with cow songs.

Thursdays are the simplest days at Folkfest. No side stages operate: only the Main Stage. I think of Thursdays as Folkfest warm-up, the night we stretch our rusty festival muscles before the sustained workout that is Friday through Sunday. On this first night, I often sit on the tarp and look out at the crowd as much as I listen to the music. I always see familiar faces, faces of people I know, might wave to. I also see faces of people I don't know, but that I've seen before, last August and the August before that. I notice that some people wear the same clothes to Folkfest each year—and wonder what I wore last year. Many carry the same chairs, sport the same packs on their backs.

Families have been created at Folkfest. It's unlikely that any babies have actually been conceived here because there is no overnight camping on site. But couples have met at Folkfest, courted there, brought their children to see the performances, watched them grow up and start the whole process over again.

Fridays are when the festival shifts into a higher gear, even though the music doesn't start until six o'clock. From six to nine, the Main Stage is quiet. The side stages come to life. For me, the smaller stages are the best part of Folkfest. Main Stage has the size and the glamour, but the other stages are where magic can happen. Three, four, or five performers and their backup bands crowd onto those smaller spaces, their audiences seated tarpless on the grass in front of them. People drift in and out on their way to and from other stages. Each performer takes a turn with a song. The others listen, perhaps join in. When they do, the session turns into jamming. Jamming results in music that hasn't been heard before and won't be heard again. Jamming can be messy, or magic, or messy magic.

On the Friday night of my distraction year, I was restless. For the first hour I drifted, walked the length of the site from Stage One on the far east to Stage Six on the far west. The sessions were everything they should be, intimate and innovative, but still I moved on. Finally, I settled at Stage Five for a solo concert by Martyn Joseph, a singer-songwriter from Wales. He'd been to Folkfest before, and I'd always found both his music and his personality appealing. As he settled himself at the microphone, I noticed that he looked older than the last time I'd seen him. The boyish charm was now accompanied by a certain weariness. His shoulders were more rounded and a few lines etched his brow. Where previously his aura had been that of an impish rebel, now it was that of a subdued guerilla leader. He looked how I felt. I listened as he talked to his audience. Martyn was in a mood to chat that evening, rambling from one topic to another, from bartenders to absent fathers to Bruce Springsteen songs.

Stage chatter is not unusual at Folkfest. Between songs, while they tune their instruments, the performers talk to their audiences as if they were sitting in a living room. Or a bar. Their comments range from the personal to the political to the philosophical. They are comic and tragic, angry and joyful. To their credit, Folkfest audiences aren't like bar audiences. In a bar, people talk incessantly between and during songs. At Folkfest, the audience, especially at the side stages, listen to the people they came to see and hear.

On Saturdays, Folkfest runs at full capacity. From eleven o'clock in the morning until well after midnight, music is in the air. We hear it everywhere we walk, and we walk a lot: back and forth from Stage One to Stage Six, up and down the small hills, up and down the big one. Walking at Folkfest is not fast and never solitary. The temporary paths are well-trodden. In wet weather, they turn into a muddy quagmire. In dry heat, they are dusty trails. When the sun beats down on Gallagher Park, we share a collective sweat, and our steps slow to a languid saunter.

By Saturday, I was feeling better, the greyness of my distraction lifting a little. That afternoon, I sat under my sun umbrella and watched a man in front of me put the flat of his hand on the small of a woman's back. Did she feel pressure or affection? Too much warmth or just the right amount of love? Beside me, I saw a young daughter, about five years old, smooth sunscreen on her mother's back. Her strokes were slow caresses that continued long after the white lotion had disappeared into her mother's skin, as if the daughter's small hands did not want to detach themselves from the body that created her. I couldn't remember ever putting sunscreen on my mother's back—or any kind of lotion for that matter. I pictured my mother's skin in the year before she died, becoming more and more translucent, until the last time I saw her I could almost see her bones.

Back on stage, Rory Block, a lanky American with waist-length brown hair, sang alone, without instrumental accompaniment—a cappella. She sang out to the rapt crowd sitting shoulder to shoulder, spreading from right in front of the stage to far up the grassy slope. She sang about the last whale on earth, a song titled "The Great Leviathan." It's a haunting lament about our planet's ultimate death, delivered as the thoughts of the last living member of a once thriving species. Her audience was still, silent, unmoving until the last faint note evaporated into the air. Then we leapt to our feet and applauded until our hands hurt.

Folkfest Sundays are wind-down days. The morning bull-pen is quieter than usual as Folkies conserve their energy for the final festival hours ahead. Sunday morning bullpens often find me grumbling that herding sleep-deprived music fans into a fenced-in enclave at seven in the morning is not an appropriate way for Folkfest organizers to treat their most loyal customers. But I'm still there.

In the early Sunday afternoon hours of my distraction year, I stood off to the side of Stage One as a big show from New Orleans entertained one of the biggest side-stage crowds of the day. Nearby, I saw a woman old enough to be called elderly. She wore a red, yellow, and black poncho with a pattern of sunbeams, stars, and crescent moons as she danced, off-beat and slowly, to the rhythm of the masterful piano blues coming from the stage. Nearby a trio of young girls swirled around, all young enough to be her granddaughters, maybe even her great-granddaughters. An hour later, I saw her again, in the middle of the kids' water-spray park, standing under the main spout, her silver hair plastered flat against her head, forehead, and cheeks. She smiled upwards, her mouth wide open to receive the wet.

At Stage Three, I listened as Johnny Clegg, an energetic performer from South Africa, chatted between songs about how seeking validation is a lifelong exercise. He said that those who are most successful at this exercise need less and less validation from established, and often disapproving, sectors. I assumed that by this, he meant that some people learn how to give themselves the validation they need. Rhythm, he continued, is time. His music was a smorgasbord of beats, from a waltz to energetic merengues. At both sides of the stage, dancers moved their bodies. They danced to their own rhythms, together but alone, with partners, friends, and strangers. I noticed one woman in particular. She was scrawny-shouldered and had one of those caved-in belly bodies. Her arms were skinny and her hands bony. Her body didn't look like it would have the capacity to move with abandon, but it did. My toes tapped on the grass as I watched her, and thought how the upbeats made both the dancing and the living easier. I became aware that my head was nodding ever so slightly in time to the music.

On Sundays, the mood is mellow. At the small side stages, those who have spent the last three days sitting forward on their haunches, leaning into the music, now lie back on the grass. Some even sleep. It's a day for Folkfest reverie. I'll lie on the hill with moments from past festivals still vivid in my mind, like the time years ago when I saw Kate and Anna McGarrigle together at Stage One. Not on the stage, but right in front of me, sitting on the grass watching their children—Rufus, Martha, and Lily—perform. Two sisters as part of an audience, two proud mothers basking in the results of their mothering.

I'll relive Laura Smith's indelible version of "My Bonny," her own original lyrics mingling with the ballad's traditional lines. It was during one of my first Folkfests, and I thought, wow, that's allowed. You can mess with what already exists, reshape it, add to it.

I'll see Mary Chapin Carpenter again, singing on the Main Stage during a drenching rainstorm. She turned her face up towards the dark grey sky as she shouted out how lucky she felt that day.

Or Brandi Carlile leading a Stage Six Sunday morning jam session in an unforgettable rendition of "Folsom Prison Blues." Johnny Cash must have smiled down from another realm that day.

And always the candles. Folkies love candles. As the sun goes down, we light up. Folkfest organizers keep us from setting each other on fire by selling protective candle holders and insisting that we use them. And we do. As a result, when darkness falls on Gallagher Park's main hill, Folkfest looks like a glowing vigil. We know this because the Main Stage performers tell us every year. When Alberta's own k. d. lang saw the candlelit hill again, decades after her first festival appearance in 1984, she said she still had no words to describe it. We held our candles higher and waved our approval.

In the year of my distraction, blues artist Bonnie Raitt brought the Festival to a close on Sunday night. For me, Folkfest isn't usually about the headliners. For me, it's been about the unknown musicians and performers I've discovered there, the people whose voices I'd bought to take home with me,

and played so often, I felt as if I knew them personally. But I'd
listened to Bonnie Raitt's music for as long as she'd been putting
it out there. For years, I'd hoped that she'd eventually come to
Folkfest. On that night, it was all about the headliner for me.
When she launched into "Something to Talk About," I jumped
to my feet. Along with everyone else on the hill, I belted out the
words. My hips swayed and my feet tapped out double time.
At one point during her set, Raitt sat on a stool and gave us her
stunning version of "I Can't Make You Love Me." I grabbed my
daughter and held her close. My husband came up behind and
put his arms around both of us.

Halfway through her set, Raitt gazed up at the flickering
mass in front of her and said, "I'm glad I'm sober." Then she
turned to her stage assistant: "Hand me that Stratocaster, baby.
I ain't foolin' around." And a voice in my head said, "Neither are
we, Bonnie. Neither are we."

The next morning, I hummed as I shook the tarp out in my
back yard, hummed as I rolled up the blue plastic and stuffed it
into its sack, hummed myself into the garage to return it to the
peg where it spends three hundred and sixty-one days each year.

Current Crossings

Edmonton's High Level Bridge is over one hundred years old. An active centenarian, this distinctive river span continues to function as a major artery, a downtown aorta all Edmontonians flow through sooner or later, a visceral element of our central core.

Begun in 1911, its construction took almost two years. Its design was innovative, accommodating streetcar, railway, motor vehicle, and pedestrian traffic. Although trains no longer travel on the bridge, people still use several different transportation modes to cross it today: they do so on foot, on bicycles, enclosed in motor vehicles, or riding a streetcar that glides along the top tier tracks. This last option is available only in the summertime.

Standing at the north or south end, the bridge's span and height disappear. It looks like a long rectangular tube propped up by the high riverbanks on both sides. It's tube-like because of the trussed canopy that elevates the train tracks above the motor vehicle and pedestrian lanes. Drivers of large trucks who ignore the bridge's height restriction warning risk seeing photos of their folly under scornful headlines in the newspapers the next day.

To fully appreciate the bridge's length and height, to observe its trestles and concrete pillars, the High Level must be seen from the east or the west, preferably from the middle of another bridge, perhaps the pedestrian level of the light rail transit (LRT) bridge beside it. But to live it, truly feel the pulse of this bridge, it must be crossed. Several times.

In the years leading up to and following my mother's death, I felt myself drawn to the bridge. It pulled me to cross it whenever I could, however I could. I still feel that attraction. While moving around the city, my eyes seek it out. If it's in my view, I will be looking at it. My feet seek it too. If I can cross it, I do.

Sometimes I cross the bridge without thinking about it. My mind is elsewhere, on what lies at my destination, on what I'll do once I get to where I'm going. At other times, I'm present in my bridge moment, aware of where I am—right in the middle of my city, far above the North Saskatchewan River.

In a car, the crossing is quick and dark. These days, motor vehicles move one-way only, a traffic pattern intended to send cars, small trucks, and buses flowing out of Edmonton's downtown core into the neighbourhoods and suburbs of south Edmonton. In the summertime, when a breeze blows through open windows, when traffic is light, when thunks from other vehicles reverberate only a few times, the crossing takes about fifty-eight seconds.

Even at noon, driving across the bridge can feel like dusk. On a long lazy summer evening, the sky will still be light, but the bridge's dark canopy will cast its ever-present shadows. The light flashing through the overhead trusses flickers across windshields like movies on fast-forward.

After four o'clock on weekday afternoons, traffic increases. Vehicles inch steadily across, drivers and passengers alike hoping that the dreaded full stop doesn't happen. Full stops mean trouble on the bridge. People will crane their necks to see where the blockage is, to guess which lane will offer the quickest exit.

When I forget what time of day it is, forget to choose an alternate late afternoon route, and find myself stuck in rush-hour traffic, I listen to the music of the bridge, to the growl of blue and silver Edmonton Transit buses in the next lane. I watch puffs of exhaust escape from their rear pipes, feel the aroma of diesel fuel seep into my nostrils. If I'm lucky and traffic doesn't come to a complete halt, this crossing takes about three and a half minutes.

As always, I watch for the spot almost halfway across where my car had a flat tire early one frosty November morning a few years ago. Refusing to succumb to that most embarrassing of Edmonton motorist moments—an emergency stop on the High Level—I kept driving until I reached Saskatchewan Drive. There I finally pulled over and stood looking at my completely shredded tire, wishing I'd stayed home in my warm bed.

Released from the confines of a motor vehicle, set free on their feet or on a bicycle, bridge-crossers experience a more immediate journey. Traffic flow expands into two directions because feet and bicycle wheels escape the two one-way vehicle lanes. Encounters that are not car accidents may happen. The pedestrian paths open up possibilities of human contact both going and coming.

Some days, when the sun is right and the wind is light, I ride my bike along River Road, cross the pedestrian path suspended under the LRT Bridge, and climb up the steep bank out of the river valley on the south side. About halfway, I usually have to get off my bike and walk the rest of the way to the top. Once my breathing settles down, I tighten my helmet and remount my bike for the northward trip across the High Level.

On a bicycle crossing, there is no time to look around, no time to take in the view, and no time to decode all the echoing sounds coming from the bridge deck. This is a focused trip. I steer carefully down through the S-turn past the iron girders, weave through pedestrian traffic while avoiding any bikes coming the other way. My left index finger is at the ready on my bell, my right-hand fingers move from the gear shift to the brake, alert for necessary quick bursts and stops, preparing for the spin out onto the north side.

Other days, when a stretch of good weather beckons me, I leave my bike at home and drive to the south side. There I park my car in a secret spot near the High Level Diner, home of the best vegetarian burger in the city. A few minutes later, I'm standing at the bridge's south end, listening to car wheels thud as they hit the seams of the bridge surface. Bigger vehicles and those going too fast generate much louder thuds. Motorcycle whines reverberate off the trusses.

I like to time my crossings and estimate that this one will take about ten minutes, depending on how long I make my stride. Running or jogging would be faster, but fast isn't the point. Fast is rarely the point for me. Making my way down onto the flat of the bridge, I'm passed by runners who thread through pedestrians, similar to the way cyclists weave through those on foot. I consider asking one runner how long it takes him to get across, but he looks very intense and unlikely to take interruption well.

I start my stopwatch and decide to count my steps as I go. On foot, everything changes. A walk across the west pedestrian lane on a summer evening is a light-filled experience. This path puts me outside the bridge's canopy, into the airspace. I stop for a moment to look to the horizon, note the yellowing of the sky's blue, assess the few dark clouds gathering in the northwest. Below me is the blue span of the LRT Bridge. I watch as a train with four white and blue cars crosses, counting the seconds as it goes. Twenty-six.

This is not a quiet walk, not conducive to a chat-filled stroll with a friend. Conversations on the High Level often go unheard, especially at rush hour. At five o'clock on a weekday afternoon, my head fills with the relentless churning of homeward-bound vehicles progressing as fast as they can towards the freedom of the south-side thoroughfares. Traffic sounds and a stiff wind batter my eardrums.

The wind is a common companion on the bridge. This high up, even a light breeze brings resistance. Stronger winds keep me close to the trusses. Whatever its strength, the wind takes up much audio space in my head. I wonder if that's why so many bridge-walkers wear earphones connected to various devices. But then again, they probably wear them when walking along sheltered, sparsely populated river valley paths.

On crossings during a light wind, I can focus on my surroundings. Ahead of me, on the north side, is the sprawling Royal Glenora Club, its parking lot fairly full. How many of those vehicle owners are inside their club, using its dining rooms, pools, and gyms? How many are outside in the river valley? How many of those cars don't belong to club members? Beyond the club, rows of high-rise condominium buildings dominate the city's skyline, their lower levels falling into shadow even as the windows on their top floors still glow orange.

Almost all the other bridge-walkers pass me, everyone except a young man wearing a green T-shirt from the University of Alberta Athletic Department. As I overtake him, I note that he is perhaps the least athletic-looking person on the bridge this evening. But then again, I can't see myself, and if I could, I wouldn't see me as others do.

I continue, still counting my steps. I've already lost track several times because it's difficult not to get distracted up here. Now halfway across, I start counting out loud, disregarding the strange looks that come my way from other bridge-users. Twice, I stop and pull out my camera to capture the sun's reflection on the river's darkening surface. When I start taking steps again, I can't remember whether I was at five hundred and fifty-six or six hundred and fifty-five. Once on the other side, my count is at one thousand and thirty-six. Or is it nine hundred and thirty-six? I settle on a thousand and pull out my stopwatch: my walk across the bridge took ten minutes and twenty-six seconds. It felt longer.

My feet take me to a bench in Ezio Faraone Park, named for an unfortunate young police officer killed while doing his job. I look back at the bridge, watching red rear lights flash between its dark girders. Looking directly south, I see the University of Alberta's main campus: visible in front of me is the stark cement bunker known as the Humanities Building, the glass dome of Hub Mall rising behind it. Nearby is the no-nonsense Henry Marshall Tory Building, with its unmistakable tall thin silhouette. The bench is a prime spot to sit and watch the evening move inevitably towards night, but my car is on the south side, so I get to my feet and begin my return crossing.

I notice that the bridge seems noisier now, even with my somewhat deaf ear now turned towards the traffic lanes. Buses rumble, several crotch-rockets roar by. On the pedestrian path, cyclists' bells ring often, warning of their presence behind me. During this crossing, I also notice that most of the human traffic on the bridge is young or youngish. The late-evening crowd is emerging for the beginning of their night. Several couples hold hands, and a few joggers scowl as they jostle to pass them. A tall slender woman gliding across on long smooth strides wears her yoga mat slung over one shoulder and a Mona Lisa smile on her face. A serious young man with long dark hair carries a tray of cupcakes in a clear plastic container. They seem to be red velvet with thick creamy icing. He never takes his eyes off them, and

I'm certain that he's going to trip over his feet at any moment. Yet, with one look at the cupcakes, I understand the attraction. I can almost taste them, their sweetness mingling with the tang of thirst on my tongue.

I count one thousand and forty-eight steps this time. I'm certain this number is more accurate than the first one because I was more focused on my return crossing. Once on the other side, I check my stopwatch and am surprised to see that this took me eleven minutes and twenty-eight seconds, a whole minute longer. It didn't feel that long.

At the south end, I emerge from the bridge deck and make the climb up the S-turn towards 109 Street. Just before crossing the railway tracks, I turn to look back. On the north side, the Legislature Building's tan sandstone facade has turned to gold. I'd take in the scene a little longer, but I've become aware of a new presence: mosquitoes. I scratch at my arms, and realize that my feet are itchy too. Perhaps they just want to turn around and do the walk again, faster this time—but that's for another day. I scurry up the rise to retrieve my illegally parked car.

A few months later, it's Thanksgiving weekend and my last chance to cross the bridge on the High Level Streetcar until next year. The streetcar is more of a novelty than a mode of transportation, a sightseeing tour on rails. Its starting and stopping points penetrate deeper into south and north Edmonton than the bridge itself. The ride from the Strathcona side on the south to the north side's turn-around near Jasper Avenue is three kilometres.

On this vivid October afternoon, my streetcar is far from full, with only five passengers, a conductor, and a driver. We all have window seats aboard the green Osaka car, #247—built in Japan in the 1920s. On the way to the start of the bridge, we pass through a tunnel that serves as a furtive graffiti art gallery. After a few moments of darkness, the streetcar rolls into an open space with two parallel tracks spreading out ahead. Here the driver brings the streetcar to a full stop. It's time for the information part of the ride. Standing in the middle of the car, wearing his 1913-style uniform, the conductor tells us that the length of the bridge is 777 metres or 2,549 feet, that it has four cement supporting piers, and that it opened to traffic on June 2, 1913. I like him. He's not overly chatty. When he finishes delivering the essential data, he steps back and leaves us to think about it.

As the streetcar begins to move again, I'm not thinking about the past hundred years. I'm thinking about the quiet. Here, on the bridge's top level, above the noisy vehicle lanes, there is silence. We glide slowly across the tracks. Above us is nothing but blue. The bridge underneath is no longer visible. A panoramic canvas spreads out in all directions—a landscape of flowing river, treed banks, and yellow leaves clinging to branches until the first stiff autumn wind rises up to blow them away.

Epilogue

Two years after my mother died, I returned to Taliesin West, the place I'd been at the moment of her death. This time, instead of touring through the building, I went on a guided walk through the landscape surrounding it. There I learned that bees love yellow, and hummingbirds love red. I learned that prickly pear cactuses are part of the cholla family, related because of their segmented structures. Some pears are a hazy purple and look like the soft pads on the bottom of a puppy's paws, but you wouldn't want to touch them. Others are spineless, without the layer of needles. Still, you wouldn't want to touch them. Their prickliness might be hidden.

Saguaros are the kings of the Arizona cacti family. They grow tall and stately, a growth that takes a long time. Their root system is shallow, largely because they grow in rock and clay. But they have an astonishing ability to shoot long root tendrils out horizontally, fifty or sixty feet. They do this as soon as they sense moisture. In the Arizona desert, when rain falls, it often arrives as torrents that start and stop in sudden bursts. Saguaros take this opportunity to suck in as much moisture as they can hold, a surprising amount. A saturated saguaro has bloated shallow ridges, far apart from each other. A thirsty saguaro has deep ridges, the spaces between them shrunken until the next desert deluge.

You'd think with such a shallow root system that saguaros would blow over in a stiff wind, but they don't. They withstand the winds because they aren't rigid. They move. Touch a fingertip to a saguaro—between the spines, definitely between the spines—with a little push and it will give. Not very much, but it will move. I have two saguaro friends near where I stay in Arizona. They sway gently in the breeze. I like to recline on my patio and watch them move against the backdrop of lime-green Palo Verde trees and azure blue sky.

Saguaros are slow growers. It takes them over two decades to gain each foot in height. Thus, for their early years, they require the protection of nurse plants. They grow near Palo Verde trees, or under the branches of triangular bursage, or beside a sturdy creosote bush. After fifty or sixty years of this nursing, some saguaros grow arms. The pattern of the arms is unique to each plant, genetic. If a saguaro's mother had three arms, it likely will too, someday.

Saguaros can achieve their stately height because of their internal structure, their firm "bones" holding them sentinel-straight for decades. They will survive many wounds, but eventually, sometimes after living as long as two hundred years, they topple to the ground. I have yet to see one in its last act of falling to the desert floor, but on my hikes I pass many of their skeletons. Their decay is a long, slow process. Time eats away at the remains until bleached long bones are the only residual hints of their former soaring selves.

The desert shows off its skeletons. On the Taliesin West tour, we walked past the remains of a fishhook barrel cactus. I could see that it had been on the ground for some time, its innards completely gone. The remains were nothing but black rubble, except for those fishhook spikes. They still looked as menacing as ever, outlasting their corporeal remains by years.

A few weeks after my return visit to Taliesin West, I was back in Canada where our testy Alberta spring had arrived. That year, my May Long weekend did not include golf. Instead, I joined my siblings at a cordial gathering, the first time we'd all been together since my mother's funeral. We went through her photographs, some of her clothes, and her jewellery. We divided up her collection of Royal Doulton figurines: her ladies, she'd called them. When we were small children, tearing through the house at breakneck speeds, Mom had often warned us about the consequences of breaking one of her ladies, a warning that didn't need words: just a tilt of her head and a waggle of her index finger.

The Doulton lady I inherited has a huge billowing skirt and an impossibly small waist. She hangs onto her brimmed bonnet as she turns away from her permanent wind. Her name is Autumn Breezes. I knew exactly where I'd put Autumn Breezes at home—in my china cabinet, right next to the green glass angel I'd given my mother almost two decades ago. Together, they remind me of the bronze statue I'd seen at Taliesin West, the one of the caped figure looking up at nothing or everything.

On the Sunday of that May Long weekend, my siblings and I also turned our attention to Mom's ashes. The blue urn that held her remains had spent the last two years in a closet at my sister's house. That day, I wore blue jeans and my lime-green raincoat, not because green had been my mother's favourite colour, but because the overcast skies threatened rain. One of my sisters carried my mother in a black shoulder tote. We went to a local park near the river and walked for about twenty minutes, until we all agreed on a spot. The bag holding Mom's ashes was made of clear, heavy-duty plastic. In fact, the plastic was so heavy-duty that it was hard to open the bag. I think one of my brothers-in-law had to slash it with a knife, but I'm not sure because I was some distance away, looking at the trees, still quite bare, or the grass, still quite brown, or the river, not still, but flowing at its leisure.

Before we began spreading, I pulled a resealable plastic sandwich bag from my coat pocket and poured some of Mom into it. After that, her five adult children passed the cylinder-shaped bag of grey ashes from one to the other. We took turns scattering my mother at the bases of bare trees, among the leaf-less bushes, around the brown grassy patches.

When it was my turn, I cradled the bag to my belly first. And I felt something break loose inside me, something that exited as a howl, a primal, visceral audible exhale.

We continued spreading until the bag was empty. After that, I felt a calm settle on me. My mother was returned to the ether, and I didn't need to go searching for her any longer.

Later that day, I put the sandwich bag and its grey powdery contents into a small pale green tin I'd found while cleaning out a closet. I don't know where it came from. I don't know what its original purpose was. A still-life drawing of two pears adorns the lid. One of the pears is golden-ripe and stands shielding the other, green and immature. The tin and its contents now live in the top drawer of my nightstand, among random items I reach for when I need them—a tape measure, some hand lotion, lug-gage tags, tickets to an upcoming theatre event, a few pens, and a notebook.

Author's Note

This book is built from observation, investigation, narrative, and many personal memories. Memories feed us, keep us connected to the places we've been and the people we've spent time with. They help us understand today in the light of yesterday, help us make choices about tomorrow. Sometimes we say things like "I remember it all too well." Sometimes we're certain about the accuracy of our memories; when we aren't, we make informed guesses, whether we realize it or not.

Memories are seductive and can be shaped to serve our present circumstances. We must be aware of this when we recall and record them. In writing this book, I've tried to be aware, endeavoured to be as authentic and realistic as possible. Nevertheless, absolute accuracy cannot be guaranteed by anyone, least of all me. Conversations in my story are recreations edited by my internal narrator. Any inaccuracies are my responsibility alone.

For research, I read books and browsed the Internet, watched videos and listened to music lyrics, went for walks and looked at the sky. Neither planned nor orderly, my process

was random and unfettered. I let it pull me at will. It is a prob-
ing that continues today, that will probably never be complete.
I soon realized that if I waited until I felt my research was
finished before I started writing, I'd be waiting for the rest of my
days. Information included in this book should not be considered comprehensive. It scratches at the surface of the topics
I touch on.

Acknowledgements

Gratitude is a good emotion, especially when the opportunity to express it publicly arises. I send my deepest gratitude to all those who helped me during the creation of *A Year of Days*. A big thank you goes to everyone on the University of Alberta Press's talented team, especially the indefatigable Peter Midgley, whose support for this project has been invaluable from the beginning. This book would not exist in its present form without the expert editorial skills of Helen Moffett. I cannot thank her enough, so I will compensate by thanking her often.

The first draft of this manuscript emerged as a result of my participation in the 2012–13 Wired Writing Studio at the Banff Centre. I am deeply indebted to my "wired" mentor, Charlotte Gill, whose notes I still carry with me. As well, one of *A Year of Days*' key essays, "Wearing Black," benefitted from my week at the Banff Centre's spring 2012 Writing With Style workshop. Thanks to Merilyn Simonds and that entire workshop group. You know who you are, you False Summitters.

My thanks also go to others who offered their insights on either the whole manuscript or parts of it—Curtis Gillespie,

Jannie Edwards, and Kath MacLean. I am also grateful to Alice Major for allowing us to use the epigraph quotation from *Memory's Daughter* (University of Alberta Press 2010).

An earlier version of the chapter "Gym Interrupted" appeared in *My Life at the Gym* (SUNY Press 2010). My thanks go to that book's editor, Jo Malin.

I also want to thank my husband and my three children. Their unfailing support gives meaning to all the days of my years.